Hot Flashes, Night Sweats, and Mood Swings, Oh My!

Every Woman's Guide to Navigating Menopause

Cecilia Baumann

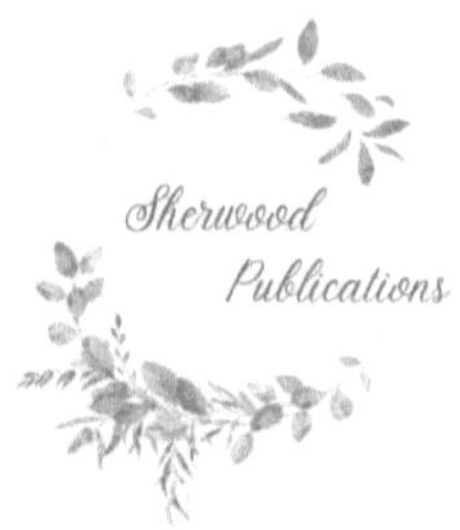

Sherwood Publications

Dedicated to all of the women on this journey.
Freedom is just ahead.

CONTENTS

Introduction
The Menopause Journey

Welcome to the carnival that is menopause! Your hormones will take roller-coaster rides, your waistline may expand in the hall of mirrors, and your moods may swing like an acrobat. You may skip periods, have no periods, have hot flashes, sleep only three hours per night, or itch and sweat all day.

In this book, we'll walk through the carnival together. We'll look at the symptoms of menopause, from the haunted house of hot flashes to the clown show of mood swings. Then, we'll walk up to each symptom and confront them head-on with facts. We'll investigate why the symptoms occur and what you can do about it. Your hormones might have put you on a carousel, but you can take control of the ride.

The first stage of the menopause carnival is called perimenopause. During perimenopause, your ovaries still produce hormones and release egg cells, but fluctuations creep in. One month you may barely have any menstrual flow, and the next might be a heavy period. You might have your first hot flash, your first night sweat, and your first proper mood swing. Your breasts might become lumpy and tender, and your sex drive may be low. Not everyone will have the same symptoms, and you may have one or two, none, or many signs of menopause. Your egg cells will get used up and your ovaries will gradually shut down.

Suddenly, there is no more estrogen or progesterone produced by your ovaries, and your periods stop forever.

Once you've been menstruation-free for a full year, you are officially menopausal. Your hot flashes may increase from a mild tropical moment to a hot lightbulb, and your waistline may expand from maidenly to matronly. The hormones that protected you against heart disease and osteoporosis are now mere trickles of their former selves, and their production has shifted to your adrenal glands, which have other things to do. Almost overnight, you might feel as if you have turned into your grandmother; your joints may ache, your knees may feel sometimes like rusty old hinges, and you may be itchy all over.

Don't despair! In this book, we'll discover exactly what happens to your body during perimenopause and menopause. You'll learn what to expect, and what you can do to make your menopause journey easier. Although the menopause journey can be a rocky one as you venture across the ocean of hormonal turmoil, you'll make it through, and sing some lovely sea shanties along the way.

This book isn't a one-size-fits-all fix. We are all different, and while some women experience the full range of menopause symptoms, some very lucky women won't have any symptoms at all, or will have only one or two mild ones. We'll discuss what you can do to relieve your symptoms—and remember, since you are unique, what works for you might not work for your sister. If one method doesn't cool your heat, soothe your skin, or pep up your sex life, try one of the other methods. **Don't give in to the symptoms, and don't give up on your bright, fulfilling future.**

We'll kick off our journey in Chapter 1 with a holistic overview of what perimenopause and menopause are, and the role of estrogen and progesterone in your physical, emotional, and mental changes. Then, in Chapter 2, we'll explore your body's secret language of signs and symptoms. **If you know what to expect, you can prepare, and if you are already experiencing the symptoms, you'll know that you aren't alone.**

The third chapter will focus on the sleepless nights of menopause. Due to hormonal imbalances, you can have difficulty falling or staying asleep, especially if you have night sweats or anxiety.

Your hair and skin change during menopause, and in Chapter 4 we'll look at what changes you can expect and what you can do to combat these changes to look and feel your best.

Chapter 5 tackles the unspoken fear of loss of libido. When sex becomes uncomfortable or painful, and we experience no sexual desire, we often keep quiet about it out of shame or fear that our partner won't understand. We fear that it could mean the end of our marriage or the end of our femininity, and, instead of seeking help, we suffer in silence. We'll investigate why your libido may take a dive and what changes the menopause brings to the vagina—and what you can do about it.

We'll follow the sexual aspects with a discussion of the emotional aspects in Chapter 6. Having mood swings, depression, or anxiety during menopause has a physical cause; the hormones that regulate your mood need estrogen to function at their best, and your estrogen levels drop dramatically as your ovaries become less active. Your body will adjust to the different hormone levels in time, but until then, there is help!

Chapter 7 is all about menopausal changes in the brain. Becoming forgetful and unfocused during this stage of your life doesn't mean you are in the first stages of a neurological disease. It is natural to have brain fog when your brain is deprived of estrogen. If you struggle with brain fog, you'll find good advice and practical steps to help you manage cognitive changes. You'll also be relieved to know that cognitive issues are temporary and, once your hormone levels stabilize, the fog will lift from your mind.

You might have heard that hormone replacement therapy (HRT) can cause cancer, or that your risk of cancer is higher if you don't have HRT. In Chapter 8, we sift through the myths and explore both HRT and natural remedies for symptom management.

Menopause changes your metabolism and may result in weight gain. The middle-age spread around the waistline doesn't occur because menopausal women can't keep their spoons out of the ice-cream bucket, but because of hormonal changes in the way they burn calories and store unburnt calories as fat. Belly fat is notoriously difficult to melt away, and in Chapter 9 we look at why women gain weight during menopause and how you can battle the bulge.

In Chapter 10, we end the book by exploring movement as medicine and how exercise can boost your energy levels naturally, and introduce a range of exercises that will limber you up, give you a boost, and bring out your inner Wonder Woman. We also take a look at how to conquer anxiety and depression through mindfulness and meditation. Reducing levels of the stress hormone cortisol will not only help ease anxiety but will also help you lose weight and focus your mind. You don't need to spend hours every day to get the benefits of stilling your mind.

Menopause is inevitable, but suffering through it is not. There are ways to deal with the symptoms to make the menopause journey as smooth as possible. Let's dive right into Chapter 1, and stare menopause in the face without fear.

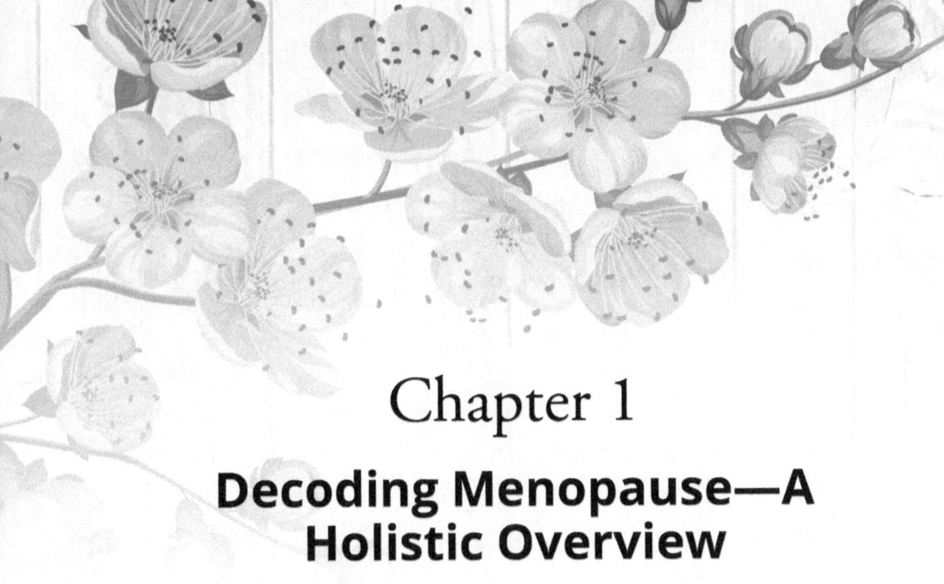

Chapter 1

Decoding Menopause—A Holistic Overview

All women will eventually experience menopause. For many of us, it will be the time when we discover just how many roles estrogen plays in our bodies, and how our bodies have to adjust to new hormone levels. The experience isn't always pleasant. There can be hot flashes, night sweats, weight gain, and hair loss. There might be sleepless nights, but unfortunately not as a result of passionate encounters but due to insomnia and night sweats.

Menopause is a natural process, but just because it is natural and inevitable doesn't mean it is insignificant. You are entering a new stage, and for the rest of your postmenopausal life you won't have another period or the same hormone levels you had during your fertile years. And, of course, you are no longer able to have a baby. It can be a big adjustment, and your body might feel like a stranger's, but it could allow you to realize a new level of freedom.

The journey starts with perimenopause. From your early 40s onward, you will notice that your periods become irregular. You might start to experience some symptoms of an imbalance between estrogen and progesterone, such as hot flashes and mood swings.

Your periods will become further apart, and you'll start skipping months until they stop completely. When you haven't had your period for a year, you are officially menopausal. Menopause happens because your ovaries have stopped releasing eggs, and production of estrogen and progesterone has shifted from your ovaries to your adrenal glands.

Because estrogen and progesterone play so many roles in your body, menopause will affect more than your reproductive system. You will have a greater risk of developing osteoporosis and cardiovascular disease, your skin might become dryer and less elastic, your metabolism can slow down, you may become prone to depression and anxiety, and you may even have days when you wonder if you are losing your mind. But rest assured, you are not. All of these symptoms are normal and natural.

With all these changes, menopause can be a confusing and challenging time. Think of it as a second puberty, in that your body is doing strange things that you have no control over. Just like in your teenage years, your hormones will be all over the place. Some symptoms of hormonal imbalance, such as memory and concentration problems, are temporary, while others, such as slower metabolism, are permanent, but they can be managed if you know how. We'll discuss the symptoms of menopause in more detail in the next chapter.

Estrogen and Progesterone

These are so much more than the hormones responsible for developing our breasts and timing our menstruation. They play an integral part in the processes whereby our bone tissue is constantly being built up and broken down, our moods are regulated, the blood flow to our brains is stimulated, our fat is distributed, our body temperature is regulated, and much more.

Before menopause, our ovaries are the main production site for estrogen and progesterone, with smaller amounts produced by the adrenal glands. After menopause, the ovaries don't produce these hormones anymore, and the small amount produced by the adrenal glands becomes the only supply depot.

Estrogen and progesterone have to be in balance for your body to function optimally. This is because the one regulates the other. This mutual regulation is especially obvious in menstruation. Estrogen facilitates the growth and thickening of the lining of the uterus, called the endometrium, while progesterone inhibits this growth to prevent cells from multiplying in an uncontrolled manner—a condition known as cancer. In the time between menstruation and ovulation, progesterone is low and estrogen levels increase, while between ovulation and menstruation the opposite is true. Thanks to this cyclical hormonal dance, your body can prepare for pregnancy and clear out the endometrium if the egg cell isn't fertilized. Estrogen and progesterone enable our entire species to continue existing.

When these hormones become imbalanced, you can have symptoms of premenstrual syndrome (PMS), where you'll feel irritable, have crying bouts, and have heavy menstrual bleeding. A severe imbalance can lead to more serious conditions, including endometriosis or polycystic ovary syndrome (PCOS).

As your ovaries become less active, your hormonal balance will be thrown off balance again, and you'll enter perimenopause. When you enter perimenopause, not only will your hormones be imbalanced, but there will be much less estrogen and progesterone in your body. The estrogen that you have in menopause is also a weaker form than the estrogen you had when your ovaries were still active.

When your estrogen levels are fluctuating or decreasing, your internal temperature goes haywire, causing the most common symptom of menopause: hot flashes. The reason for this is that estrogen and progesterone influence your core body temperature, the production of internal heat, and your body's heat dissipation ability. Every woman will experience hot flashes differently. The intensity, frequency, and duration of menopausal hot flashes are unique to every individual.

To illustrate this individual effect, let's compare the hot flashes of two sisters, Jane and Sarah. Jane started experiencing mild hot flashes at age 48 that would last for a minute or two, causing her only slight discomfort. Just a mild tropical moment, barely noticeable. However, Sarah began having intense hot flashes at age 50 that could last up to 10 minutes and leave her drenched in sweat with her skin completely flushed. Although the cause of hot flashes is the same, the experience of them can vary significantly.

Hormonal Imbalance

The gradual shutting down of your ovaries will throw your hormones off balance. This imbalance can worsen if you exercise excessively, are on a severely restrictive or unhealthy diet, or are taking certain medications. You can also develop an imbalance between your estrogen and progesterone if you have any of these conditions:

- obesity
- chronic kidney disease
- PCOS
- Turner's syndrome
- surgical removal of the ovaries
- premature ovarian failure (when the ovaries slow down or stop working before age 40)
- chemotherapy or radiation treatment
- disorders of the thyroid or pituitary glands
- severe stress
- insulin resistance

Estrogen Dominance

When your estrogen levels are consistently higher than your progesterone levels, you are considered estrogen dominant. This condition can cause or exacerbate the below:

- HR-positive breast cancer
- PCOS
- endometriosis
- uterine cancer
- uterine fibroids
- headaches
- insomnia
- breast tenderness
- loss of libido
- fatigue
- fibrocystic breast lumps
- weight gain
- bloating
- memory problems
- mood changes
- changes in the amount and frequency of menstrual bleeding
- changes in the timing of the menstrual cycle
- PMS

Progesterone Dominance

On the other hand, if your progesterone is higher than your estrogen, you can experience the following symptoms:

- mood changes

- fatigue
- skipped or delayed menstrual periods

Hormone Replacement Therapy

Menopause symptoms can be pharmaceutically treated with HRT, if you choose this route. In earlier times when only estrogen was given, women were more at risk of developing breast and uterine cancer. Nowadays, estrogen is combined with progesterone, which greatly reduces this risk.

Replenishing your estrogen and progesterone with HRT can have these effects on your menopause symptoms:

- relieves hot flashes and night sweats
- stimulates a healthy libido
- relieves vaginal dryness
- regulates mood
- increases metabolism
- maintains and stimulates optimal brain function
- maintains healthy cholesterol levels
- maintains the elasticity of heart and blood vessels
- combats bone loss

Estrogen-Only HRT

Because taking estrogen-only HRT can increase the risk of uterine cancer, this type of HRT is only prescribed for women who've had a hysterectomy (surgical removal of the uterus). Estrogen pills and injections have a higher risk of negative side effects than locally applied estrogens such as vaginal creams.

Progesterone-Only HRT

Progestin is the synthetic progesterone used for HRT. This type of HRT is prescribed for women who still have a uterus, have adverse effects when they take estrogen, or can't take estrogen due to certain medical conditions. Progestin is also suitable for women who have conditions such as PCOS or who have experienced miscarriages resulting from low progesterone levels.

However, there are side effects to progestin, including

- high blood pressure
- low blood sugar
- bloating
- mood changes
- bleeding between periods
- tender breasts
- headaches

Combined Estrogen and Progesterone HRT

This combination is ideal for women who have a uterus. It provides all the benefits of estrogen without the increased risk of uterine cancer, since progestin has a protective effect on the uterine lining.

Ideally, combined HRT should be taken only at low doses over a short time. This is to lower the risk of combined HRT causing conditions such as

- breast cancer
- uterine cancer
- stroke and blood clots (the risk increases for smokers)

Lifestyle for Hormonal Balance

There are several things you can do to promote hormonal balance naturally. If you incorporate these factors into your everyday life, you might have less of a roller-coaster ride during menopause.

Avoid Xenoestrogens

A xenoestrogen is an environmental chemical that mimics natural estrogen. These chemicals are found in plastics and personal care products. Examples of xenoestrogens are bisphenol A, polychlorinated biphenyls, and phthalates.

Reduce Inflammation

By adding turmeric, ginger, or foods rich in omega-3 fatty acids—such as fatty fish, olives, coconut oil, and eggs—to your diet, you'll lower inflammation levels and promote hormonal balance. Processed foods, sugar, and grains are inflammatory and should be eaten minimally.

Long-term inflammation, called chronic inflammation, puts stress on your body, and stress can throw your hormones out of sync. If you have any of the following signs, which can indicate chronic inflammation, speak to your doctor, nutritionist, or pharmacist about ways in which you can reduce inflammation:

- high blood sugar
- cardiovascular disease
- allergies
- chronic pain
- weight gain

- excessive belly fat
- insulin resistance or insensitivity
- inflammatory bowel disease (IBD)
- autoimmune disease

Exercise Regularly

Weight-bearing exercises will not only prevent the muscle loss associated with aging but will also improve your metabolism, since muscle burns calories. Your bone density will benefit from weight-bearing exercise, which will reduce your chance of developing osteoporosis. Menopausal loss of estrogen means your heart has lost one of its best protectors against cardiovascular disease. Regularly doing aerobic exercises will help promote heart health and also support weight management.

Pamper Your Intestines

Even your intestines are affected by the loss of estrogen. Because our intestines are where nutrients and water are absorbed, any change in the intestine can make a difference in how our body feeds itself. There are special beneficial bacteria living in your gut, called the microbiome. These tiny organisms send chemical communication signals to your immune system and brain.

During menopause, your internal microbiome also changes, leading to digestive symptoms such as diarrhea, constipation, and bloating. If you don't take extra care of your digestive health during menopause, these symptoms can worsen, and your immune system and brain can also be affected.

Pamper your gut biome by eating organic plant-based foods and fermented foods such as sauerkraut and kimchi. Make sure you stay hydrated to help your intestines digest and absorb nutrients, and fuel your microbiome with prebiotics and probiotics.

Prebiotics are foods that support your microbiome, such as dietary fiber, oats, fruits, and garlic. Probiotics are living micro-organisms that are good for your digestive system, and they'll fit right in with the organisms already in your microbiome. Eating yogurt and other bacteria-fermented foods will supplement your microbiome in a tasty way.

Maintain Your Weight

Because estrogen plays a role in where fat gets distributed, the lower estrogen levels of menopause affect where our fat goes. Our breasts become more fatty and our bellies grow. Belly fat is a serious health risk because it isn't just beneath your skin but also around the organs in your abdomen. This abdominal fat that blankets your internal organs is called visceral fat, and if you have large amounts of it, you are at higher risk of the following conditions:

- fatty liver disease
- high blood sugar
- type 2 diabetes
- a high fat concentration in your blood
- stroke
- cardiovascular disease
- sleep apnea
- high blood pressure
- colon, kidney, pancreatic, and endometrial cancer

If you are overweight or concerned about your belly fat, you should manage your weight with a healthy diet and regular exercise. Although belly fat is notoriously stubborn, it will shrink if you are determined and consistent with a healthy lifestyle.

Keep Stress to a Minimum

Stress isn't just meeting a deadline at work or being stuck in traffic. The wrong diet, sleep deprivation, and excessive stimulation all cause your body to release the stress hormones cortisol and adrenalin (epinephrine). The flood of stress hormones has a domino effect on all your hormones and can make your menopausal imbalances worse.

Avoid extra stress on your body by

- getting enough sleep. If you have insomnia or night sweats as menopause symptoms, sleep can be difficult. Speak to your doctor or pharmacist about a sleep aid that will be effective and safe for you.
- not overdoing exercise. Intense and excessive exercise will put your body under stress, and the stress hormone response will lead to belly fat digging in even more.
- reducing sugar and flour. When you eat sugary and floury foods, your blood sugar levels spike. To counteract this, your body will release more insulin. Your blood sugar will then fall rapidly, and this will signal your body to release cortisol.

Aim for Quality Sleep

Switch off your computer, TV, or phone before bed. If you keep tempting yourself to watch one more program, check one more email, or spend just half an hour more on social media, you'll never get the sleep you need. Drinking too much caffeinated coffee or energy drinks will also keep you up. If you are too wound up before bed, try relaxing yoga stretches, deep breathing exercises, meditation, or listening to soothing music to help shut down your overactive thoughts.

Consume Phytoestrogens

These are plant estrogens that you can incorporate into your diet. They will boost your estrogen levels naturally. Foods containing phytoestrogens include flaxseeds, soy, tofu, and chickpeas.

Schedule Regular Check-Up Screenings

Early detection is imperative for certain health conditions. The sooner your doctor can diagnose cancer, high blood pressure, osteoporosis, or high blood sugar, the sooner treatment can start—and the quicker you can get treatment, the better the outcomes will be. Have yourself tested regularly for breast and uterine cancer, and have your blood pressure and blood sugar checked too.

Key Takeaways

The menopause journey starts with perimenopause, when your ovaries become less active and your hormones start becoming imbalanced. Eventually, your ovaries will shut down their production of estrogen and progesterone and you'll have some of the typical symptoms of menopause, such as hot flashes, insomnia, and weight gain. You can treat the symptoms with hormone therapy, supplements, natural remedies, and lifestyle changes, all of which we'll explore in more detail as the book progresses.

Let's move on to explore the signs and symptoms of menopause. If you know what to expect from menopause, you can face the symptoms fearlessly with a plan of action to manage the symptoms.

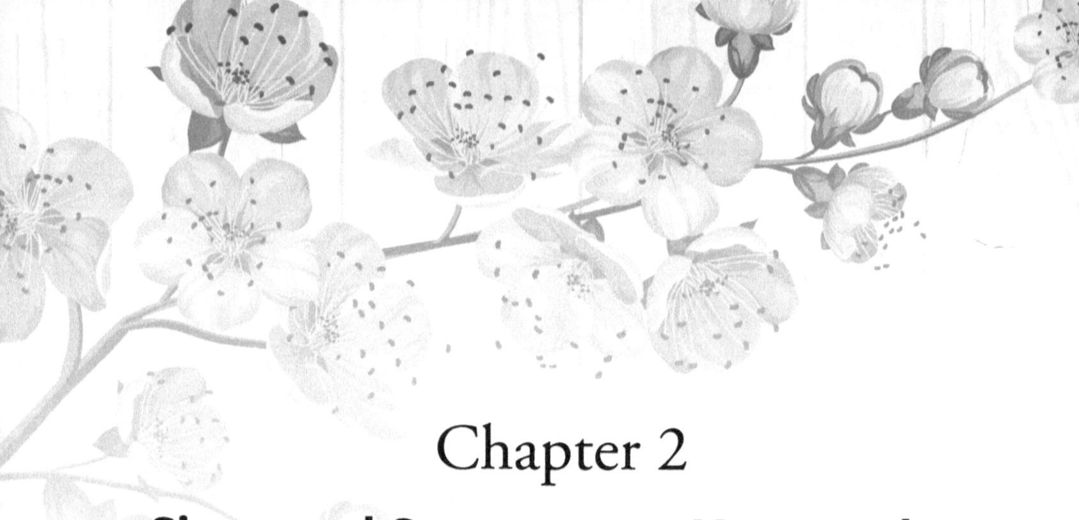

Chapter 2

Signs and Symptoms—Your Body's Secret Language

*A*s women, we are intimately aware of our bodies. We are aware of changes in our breasts before menstruation and during pregnancy, and many of us have experienced bloating and lumps, cramps, and moodiness. Our bodies talk to us all the time, and menopause is no exception. Let's take a look at the changes you can expect during menopause.

Physical Changes

Due to hormonal changes, you may gain weight, grow facial hair, and perspire even in the depths of winter. It is normal to gain about 5 pounds during menopause. All of these symptoms, and more, are signs that you are entering a new phase of your life, with new challenges, new adventures, and new opportunities for growth.

Your ovaries produce the main female sex hormones estrogen and progesterone. As you get older, your ovaries become less active and the production of these hormones starts to fluctuate. Your periods become irregular. Some months you feel like you are going to bleed to death for 10 days nonstop, and other months you could barely have a drop. These menstrual surprises could continue until your periods stop altogether.

Once you haven't had a period for a year, you are officially menopausal. You may have all kinds of uncomfortable symptoms, which will taper off gradually. Below are some of the things you can expect during menopause.

Hot Flashes

You can feel as if your face, neck, and upper chest are on fire. You might go red in your face, and sweat might pour down your body. This fiery phenomenon is caused by your estrogen embarking on a roller-coaster ride and taking the part of the brain responsible for thermoregulation with it. Hot flashes can also be triggered by exercise, drinking coffee, feeling strong emotions, or being under stress.

Hot flashes have the habit of attacking when you want them the least. I know, from personal experience. I was attending a conference and asked the speaker a question. Then, it happened. A volcano erupted in my hormones. I felt that surely everyone could see my head pulsating and glowing like a huge light bulb. The embarrassment added fuel to the fire, and the light bulb became a flaming torch that felt like it could light up the entire city.

Night Sweats

This is the twin sister of the hot flash. You might be exhausted after a day running with no estrogen in your tank and fall into bed, ready for a blissful sleep. You may still be drifting off into dreamland when your sheets turn into rivers. Night sweats can make you feel as if you are overheating in the bowels of hell, only to get the chills seconds after—and the wet sheets won't make that experience more comfortable. Thankfully, most of us won't have to change sheets in the middle of the night, but you may need to be prepared and also warn your partner if you sleep in the same bed.

Thinning Hair

I spent most of my life thinking that only men lose their hair. Don't be surprised if your once plentiful, thick tresses turn into thin, limp little stragglers and your forehead starts growing further back. A little bald patch on the crown of your head might appear. Menopause teaches you that female pattern baldness is a thing.

Dry Skin

Have you ever wondered why older women always have skin cream in their handbags? Not discreet sample-size cream, but the big bottles for extra-dry skin? Now you know. Without your regular estrogen fix, your skin can dry out and become itchy and flaky. Skin cream helps, but only if you keep slathering it on several times a day.

Loss of Libido

You might not feel sexy anymore, and your significant other may suddenly have the sex appeal of cold rice pudding. When you do muster up the energy and the drive for a naughty night, the symptoms of vaginal dryness and vaginal discomfort during sex can give you a headache. Speaking of headaches, hormonal fluctuations can easily give you a migraine.

Weight Gain

It's common to gain weight during menopause, especially around the belly, hips, and thighs. You might turn from fab to flab, and then discover that your new menopausal belly fat refuses to leave. You can't eat as much as you did before menopause, because your metabolism has slowed down to a snail's pace and your body can't burn calories like in the good old days. And all of the old tricks to stay slim don't seem to work anymore. A menopausal woman can go up a dress size by merely thinking about chocolate.

Breast Changes

Your breast glands naturally shrink due to lower estrogen levels while your breasts become more full of fat. Your nipples can become sore and your breasts could feel tender and uncomfortable. These new fatty breasts can sag and might feel itchy. Your breasts can be larger and lumpier, and noncancerous cysts aren't uncommon. On the positive side, your man may be very interested in your new larger breasts!

Joint Pain

Estrogen helps control inflammation. Without it, you'll discover that estrogen was the reason you were able to get up without your knees creaking in torment. Your shoulder joints, elbows, hands, and neck may ache constantly, and you long for the good old days when you could walk to your front door without feeling like you are about to fall apart.

Urinary Incontinence

Without wonderful estrogen, your pelvic muscles can become weaker. Among the muscles that are now too lazy to do their jobs properly are those that support the urethra and the bladder. As a result, you may embarrassingly pee when you sneeze, laugh, or even breathe too hard.

Insomnia

It is difficult to get a full night's sleep if you have night sweats and hot flashes, tender breasts, itchy skin, and aching joints. Not sleeping enough can leave anyone feeling cranky and unfocused the next day.

Emotional Changes

Anxiety and Depression

Although it hasn't been scientifically proven, most menopausal women can testify that tear ducts are affected by hormones. You may cry over everything and nothing. Seeing a dry leaf in the road will overwhelm you with a mixture of existential sadness and angst, and the tears will flow. Buttering a slice of toast will make you feel unworthy, fat, and unwanted, and the tears will flow even more. Your brain will adapt to lower hormone levels, but before then, you might experience more anxiety than a teenager on a first date.

Mood Swings

There's a reason why small children are more likely to listen to grandma than to mom. Grandma is probably menopausal, and her mood can turn on a dime. She'll lovingly hand out candy, and an instant later decide to chase children off her lawn with a frying pan. A minute later she'll be in tears, or ask for a cup of tea. Her instability makes her formidable, in an endearing way.

Cognitive Changes

Focus, Brain Fog, and Concentration

Estrogen stimulates blood flow in the brain. After your ovaries shut down their estrogen production, your brain will mourn the loss by making it difficult to concentrate. If menopause also gives you insomnia, expect to be fuzzy the next day.

You may find yourself standing in front of your fridge, wondering what you came into the kitchen for. You may have endless, fruitless searches for your keys, glasses, phone, and underwear. Then, one day, the missing objects will appear in the most obvious of places, where you forgot to look. Don't worry—you aren't losing your mind, only your estrogen.

The reason for these cognitive changes is twofold. Firstly, the loss of estrogen affects how brain cells connect with each other. Secondly, menopausal changes cause a lower level of glucose in the brain. Your brain uses glucose as fuel, and when the fuel supply starts diminishing, your brain has to adapt, which takes time. Your brain will adapt to the new low estrogen and glucose, and the fog will lift. Don't worry when you struggle to find the word for that thing you stir your coffee with, or can't remember what you had for breakfast. It is natural and temporary.

It Isn't Always Menopause

The symptoms described in this chapter are not always due to menopause. Joint pain, urinary incontinence, depression, and brain fog might have other causes. There are some illnesses that can have similar symptoms to menopause, such as post-traumatic stress disorder, low blood sugar, diabetes, tuberculosis, fibromyalgia, and urinary tract infections.

Mention all your symptoms, no matter how insignificant they might seem, to your health-care provider to make sure that any medical disorders are caught early and treated effectively.

Key Takeaways

It is impossible to predict what symptoms you may have when you are perimenopausal or menopausal. It is easy to feel overwhelmed when your symptoms affect you physically, emotionally, and cognitively, but there is help available. Also, rest assured that the symptoms are temporary, and when your body has adjusted to your lower estrogen levels, your mood will be calmer and your mind less foggy. However, you'll still be at a greater risk of developing ailments such as cardiovascular disease and osteoporosis and will have to take care of your diet and exercise to keep your risk to a minimum.

In the next chapter, we'll tackle insomnia and night sweats. We'll look at the causes, symptoms, and treatments to help you enjoy a full night of restorative sleep.

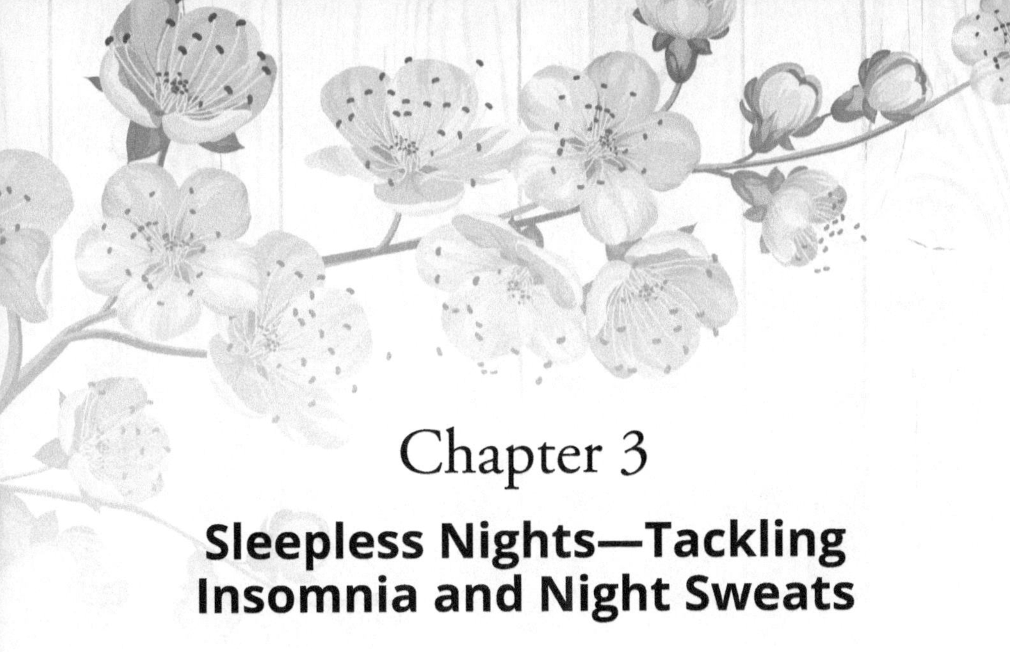

Chapter 3

Sleepless Nights—Tackling Insomnia and Night Sweats

The term "night sweats" is an accurate description of this menopause symptom. You wake up drenched, and your pajamas and sheets are almost dripping with sweat. This can occur even in the dead of winter and may happen more than once per night.

During the night, your blood vessels may expand suddenly, and this results in an increased blood flow. During the few moments or minutes when this increased blood flow is occurring, you sweat and your skin becomes flushed. You may also experience heart palpitations. Afterward, your blood vessels contract again, and you might feel chilled. Night sweats are not exactly the same as hot flashes. While a hot flash may not necessarily make you sweat, a night sweat certainly will, and the latter usually last longer than a hot flash.

The severity and duration varies from woman to woman. Having night sweats, even if they are mild, can exacerbate the insomnia that many women experience due to hormonal changes.

What Causes Night Sweats?

The hypothalamus region of the brain is the control headquarters for several bodily functions. It regulates your internal thermostat, determines if you should feel hungry or thirsty, and signals the pituitary gland to release hormones. It depends on hormones to keep it up to date about the state of your body, and if your estrogen and progesterone levels fluctuate, the hypothalamus can't get accurate information and the regulatory system gets confused.

If you have night sweats, it might not be from menopause; there are several conditions and side effects of medications that can cause this symptom. Just to be on the safe side, consult your health-care provider to rule out any of these medical conditions:

- lupus
- gastroesophageal reflux disease (GERD)
- obstructive sleep apnea
- tuberculosis
- HIV/AIDS
- diabetes
- cancer

You can also have night sweats as a side effect of any of these medications:

- antidepressants
- aromatase inhibitors
- medication to treat high blood pressure
- steroids
- diabetes medication
- tamoxifen
- opioids

Treatment for Hormonal Night Sweats

Night sweats can start during your perimenopause and can carry on for years. It isn't unusual to have night sweats for more than a decade. Fortunately, there is help.

The standard pharmaceutical treatment is HRT or, if you can't or prefer not to use HRT, Brisdelle (paroxetine).

You can also make lifestyle changes to help manage night sweats. Let's take a look at what you can do to relieve your night sweats naturally.

Avoiding Triggers

Certain foods or beverages cause chemical reactions that confuse your internal thermostat, resulting in a hot flash or night sweats. For this reason, it is better to steer clear of spicy foods, alcohol, or caffeine close to bedtime. If you smoke, quit—or at least don't smoke close to bedtime since this can also trigger night sweats. Exercise helps to reduce night sweats and hot flashes, but if you exercise too close to bedtime, your body temperature will be higher than usual, which might trigger night sweats.

Slowing Your Breathing

Simply slowing down your breathing to a rate of six to eight breaths per minute can relieve the severity and amount of hot flashes and night sweats. Ideally, you should do the slow breathing twice daily for 15 minutes at a time. When a hot flash or night sweat starts, you can slow your breathing to get relief.

Meditation

Being relaxed can help ease night sweats and hot flashes. One of the easiest ways to relax your body and mind is by meditation. When you meditate, your parasympathetic nervous system can be activated, which triggers deep relaxation.

Cardio Exercises

Doing sustained activities such as walking or jogging can reduce night sweats and hot flashes. A study found that menopausal women who joined a 16-week cardio exercise program had improved thermoregulatory control, meaning they had fewer hot flashes and stayed cooler for longer (Bailey et al., 2016).

Strength Training

A study on postmenopausal women with moderate and severe hot flashes and night sweats showed that resistance training (working out with weights or resistance bands) reduced the frequency of internal heat waves. The women reported that they had half the amount of night sweats and hot flashes they used to have after 15 weeks of strength training (Berin et al., 2019).

Soy

Some plants are rich sources of a type of estrogen called isoflavones. Soy is one of these isoflavone sources, and one of the isoflavones in soy, called daidzein, is changed by your intestinal bacteria into equol.

Equol can reduce the frequency and intensity of hot flashes and night sweats. Some dietary sources of soy include soy milk, tofu, edamame, and miso.

Black Cohosh

This plant is native to North America and, although it can't take hot flashes and night sweats away completely, it can make them less frequent and reduce their intensity. Check with your doctor or pharmacist before taking a black cohosh supplement, because you might experience side effects or interactions with medication.

Flaxseeds

Flaxseeds contain lignans, which can help balance your hormones. The more your hormones are on an even keel, the less you'll experience hot flashes and night sweats.

Wild Yam

Certain kinds of wild yam are sources of plant estrogens, also known as phytoestrogens. One of these phytoestrogens in wild yam, called diosgenin, is used to make synthetic estrogen and progesterone for HRT. Changing diosgenin to estrogen and progesterone takes many steps in a lab, and it isn't certain if the human body can also change diosgenin into estrogen.

Despite the lack of evidence, wild yam is still a popular natural remedy for night sweats and hot flashes. Wild yam products are used to relieve not only night sweats and hot flashes but also vaginal dryness and loss of libido.

Room Temperature

If you sleep in a room that is as cool as you can comfortably manage, you will have less chance of experiencing night sweats. If you do have a hot flash or night sweats, you can have a few sips of ice-cold water to help cool you down. Also, avoid wearing heavy, tight, or warm pajamas, and consider investing in sheets or mattresses that contain special cooling gels or fibers.

Sleep Deprivation

Not getting enough deep, quality sleep can cause you to be drowsy during the day, and can influence your mood and ability to concentrate. If your night sweats become so intrusive on your sleep pattern that they affect your everyday life, it is time to see your doctor.

You should also consult a health-care professional if you are having night sweats that are accompanied by coughing, diarrhea, pain, fever, and unexplained weight loss, since this might indicate another health problem that needs treatment.

Key Takeaways

It is natural to experience drenched nights during menopause. Although it is everything but comfortable, it won't affect your overall health except if it deprives you of sufficient sleep. Fortunately, there are several things you can do to reduce night sweats, from HRT to changing your lifestyle and taking supplements.

Join me in the next chapter for an in-depth look at what happens to your physical appearance during menopause, when your beauty transitions to a more mature look, and what you can do to manage the change in your skin and hair.

Chapter 4

Beauty in Transition—Coping With Skin and Hair Changes

Kate isn't vain, or a beauty queen, but she's always taken care of her appearance and is proud of looking neat and professional at work. She never leaves the house without makeup and has her hair done once a month. Kate didn't expect that being perimenopausal would affect her skin and hair since she takes good care of herself. But, despite using moisturizer daily and conditioning her hair after each shampoo, her skin is much drier and her hair less lustrous than a year ago. She doesn't want to admit it to herself, but she has also noticed her skin getting fine lines and a bit of looseness in the jowls.

Many women find themselves in Kate's position. They feel unprepared for menopausal changes in appearance and don't know how to manage them. This can lead to a drop in self-esteem and self-confidence, and even depression when the reflection in the mirror feels like the face of a stranger.

Although age is inevitable and menopause can result in changes in appearance, you don't have to throw your moisturizer and hairbrush away in despair. You can adapt to these natural changes and keep your hair and skin healthy and looking good. Aging gracefully is simply accepting change and enjoying an appearance that has a larger emphasis on elegance and alluring maturity.

The changes of menopause can be visibly seen in the skin and hair. Hormonal shifts lead to changes in skin elasticity and hydration, and hair can thin out and break more easily. In this chapter, we'll discover what changes menopause can bring to your appearance and how you can keep control of your looks. Sometimes, the key to beauty can be as simple as avoiding harsh chemicals and being aware of and prepared for changes in your body chemistry.

To know how to keep our skin healthy and looking good, we first need to understand what skin is.

Skin

Your skin is your largest sensory organ. It has sensors to tell your brain information about temperature, pressure, pain, and humidity. The sweat glands in your skin are necessary for body temperature regulation, and your skin is your first line of defense against disease-causing organisms in the environment.

Layers of the Skin

Epidermis

Skin is made up of three layers. The outermost part is called the epidermis and its thickness varies according to where on the body it is. Your thinnest epidermis is found on your eyelids, and the thickest on the soles of your feet and the palms of your hands. Conditions such as acne, dandruff, and eczema affect the epidermis.

There is much more to the epidermis than merely an outside

covering that can get pimples. It consists of five sub-layers, which each its own role in skin elasticity, hydration, and waterproofing. The outermost layer helps to lock moisture in your skin, and underneath that is a layer that facilitates skin stretching. Moisture content and elasticity are very important for skin that appears fresh, smooth, and healthy.

Dermis

This is the skin's middle layer. It consists of connective tissue such as collagen and elastin, capillary blood vessels, hair follicles, and nerve endings. The dermis is also where you'll find the glands that produce sweat and oil. The skin conditions that can affect the dermis are sun damage, collagen disorders, hives, and tumors.

The dermis isn't a continuous block of skin but has two sub-layers, which sense delicate touch, pressure, and vibration.

Hypodermis

This innermost layer is also called the subcutaneous layer and is where most of our body fat is stored. This fat is needed to insulate us against temperature changes and to protect our internal organs and muscles from impact. The hypodermis can be affected by conditions such as tumors, hypothermia, bedsores, and third-degree burns.

Collagen

Collagen is a protein needed for so many things that it is the most common protein in your body. Like every protein, collagen is made up of amino acids. To form collagen, amino acids come together to form a triple helix of protein fibrils.

In the skin, collagen facilitates the growth of new skin cells in the dermis (the middle layer of the skin), helps in the replacement of dead skin cells, and provides structure and elasticity to the skin. Collagen also forms a protective layer around organs, plays a part in the clotting of blood, and gives structure to bones, ligaments, and tendons.

In cosmetology, collagen injections are used as dermal fillers to reduce wrinkles and lines. Several skin creams contain collagen, and you can also take collagen supplements.

Elastin

Elastin is the special protein that gives our skin the ability to stretch and then reform to its original shape. It is much more flexible than collagen and is found in the skin, blood vessels, and lungs—all organs that need to be flexible and to expand and contract. If your elastin gets damaged, you'll have visible fine lines, frown lines, smile lines, thin skin, loose skin, saggy skin, and wrinkles.

If you have damaged elastin, you can repair the damage to some extent and prevent further damage by taking an antioxidant supplement, keeping hydrated, quitting smoking, exercising, and using moisturizers or skin serums that contain vitamins A, C, and E.

Skin Changes

As we age, our bodies produce less collagen, the collagen we do have breaks down faster, and the quality of our collagen deteriorates. Menopause will also contribute to a decline in collagen production.

Although there isn't a blood test to see how much collagen you have and whether your levels are dropping, there are symptoms that show your collagen levels are falling, such as

- ligaments and tendons become stiffer
- cartilage becomes worn out, leading to osteoarthritis and painful joints
- weakened or achy muscles
- wounds take longer to heal
- facial features become hollow, especially around the eyes
- wrinkly and saggy skin
- dry skin
- skin becomes less elastic
- thinner skin

How to Protect Your Skin

To make the triple helix of protein that is collagen, your body needs the amino acids hydroxyproline, proline, and glycine, as well as manganese, copper, vitamin C, and zinc. Keep an eye on your diet or supplements to make sure you are providing your body with these ingredients. You can include mushrooms, egg whites, cabbage, and wheat in your diet to provide proline; red meats, granola, and poultry to provide glycine; and fruits and vegetables for vitamin C. To provide copper, eat nuts, seeds, leafy green vegetables, liver, and dark chocolate; and consume red meat, poultry, dairy products, and leafy greens for zinc. You will find manganese in foods such as shellfish, spinach, black tea, and chickpeas.

Because smoking damages elastin and collagen, smokers tend to have more saggy, wrinkly skin. This effect on the skin is caused by the action of nicotine, which narrows the blood vessels at the skin's surface. This narrowing means that less oxygen and nutrients can make it through, and this deprivation will show as dull, crepey skin. If you are a smoker, the best way to improve your skin and reduce wrinkles is to quit.

Don't spend long periods outside in the sun, and use sunscreen or long-sleeved clothes and a wide-brimmed hat to prevent sun damage to your skin. However, because your skin needs some sunshine to make vitamin D, you shouldn't avoid the sun altogether.

Collagen can become weak and brittle when it gets damaged by sugar attached to certain proteins. To avoid this damage, limit your intake of carbohydrates and sugar.

Excessive alcohol use can cause your body's natural collagen production to slow down, causing your skin to age faster.

Stay away from processed foods and high-sugar foods, since they will stimulate a process called glycation. Glycation has a negative effect on your collagen turnover and prevents collagen from interacting properly with cells.

Stick to a good skincare routine. Don't go to bed with your makeup on, because this can lead to clogged pores, which is a one-way ticket to skin breakouts. Washing your face once daily is usually enough, but you can wash twice a day if you have oily skin. If you go overboard with the cleansing and wash your face more than twice daily, you will make wrinkles and fine lines worse because you'll strip your skin of the natural oils needed to keep the skin supple.

Be gentle on the skin around your eyes. If you manhandle this delicate skin with pulling, tugging, or pressing, you can end up with fine lines and unattractive broken blood vessels. Try not to rub your eyes hard with your hands, and put a damp cloth on your eyes instead if they feel itchy or tired.

How to Improve Skin Elasticity

Retinol and Retinoids

Retinol, which is a form of vitamin A, is an ingredient of some over-the-counter (OTC) facial and eye serums and creams. It helps restore skin elasticity and is especially effective when it is used in combination with vitamin C.

Retin-A and tretinoin are retinoids that are only available by prescription. They are more effective than OTC retinol products and are especially good at reversing the effects of skin aging due to sun exposure.

Witch Hazel

Witch hazel is a well-known and trusted ingredient in several skin-care products. There are several varieties of witch hazel, of which *Hamamelis virginiana* is the most potent remedy to restore skin elasticity and firmness and minimize wrinkles.

Pantothenic Acid

Pantothenic acid, also called dexpanthenol, is available as a moisturizer called pantoderm. This cream will reduce skin dryness and roughness, and can preserve the skin's elasticity.

Collagen Supplements

Taking a collagen supplement, especially in combination with vitamin

C, can replenish your skin's collagen, resulting in smoother, firmer skin with improved elasticity. You can also get collagen by drinking bone broth, which is made with fish or poultry bones, skin, and ligaments.

Make sure you provide your body with amino acids, which are the components of proteins such as collagen. Eat plenty of protein-abundant foods such as beans, eggs, and meats. Also, take a vitamin C supplement or eat foods abundant in vitamin C, such as berries and citrus fruits.

Many collagen supplements contain collagen in hydrolyzed form. Hydrolyzed collagen refers to collagen that is broken down into smaller bits that your body can absorb more easily.

As an extra bonus, your bone health can improve if you take a collagen supplement. This is because collagen forms part of the bone matrix, in which calcium and other minerals are laid down.

It is very unlikely that you'll have any side effects from a collagen supplement, unless your supplement combines collagen with other substances.

HRT

An estrogen cream, patch, or pill will replace the estrogen lost during menopause. Since estrogen activates the cells that make collagen, menopause can contribute to lowered collagen production, which leads to wrinkly skin.

Taking estrogen can help your skin in numerous ways:

- increasing skin thickness
- reducing the appearance of deep wrinkles
- stimulating faster wound healing
- improving skin hydration
- improving skin rigidity, which will decrease sagging

Hyaluronic Acid

Hyaluronic acid is responsible for helping your skin retain moisture. If you spend long periods in the sun without sunscreen, the ultraviolet rays can harm the hyaluronic acid in the connective tissue. This will dry out the skin and make it less elastic. Replenish your hyaluronic acid with a cream or serum to help your skin regain elasticity.

Cocoa Flavanols

By eating chocolate, especially dark chocolate with a high cocoa flavanol content, you can regain some skin elasticity and smooth the appearance of wrinkles. You can indulge in chocolate without guilt since it is part of your skin rejuvenation routine!

Genistein Isoflavones

Phytoestrogens are substances in plants that mimic the action of estrogen in your body. Soy is abundant in a certain phytoestrogen called genistein isoflavone. A study has shown that genistein isoflavones speed up wound healing and make the skin thicker and more elastic (Irrera et al., 2017).

Platelet-Rich Plasma Injections

Platelet-rich plasma (PRP) therapy uses ingredients in your own blood to stimulate cell growth. The first step of this treatment involves having a small amount of blood drawn, which is then spun in a centrifuge to separate the blood components. The PRP that will be used for your skin thus consists of your own blood platelets, stem cells, and growth factors. This specially concentrated plasma will then be injected into your skin to stimulate collagen formation. The new collagen will improve skin elasticity and firm up the skin. PRP also reduces puffiness under the eyes.

PRP injections can only be performed by nurse practitioners, registered nurses, medical doctors, physician's assistants, dentists, osteopathic doctors, and oral surgeons.

Laser Treatment

Your skin contains water molecules, which vaporize surrounding skin cells when heated up with a laser. When the cells are vaporized, a process called fibroplasia starts, which triggers the production of fresh collagen. This will result in smoother, tighter, and less wrinkly skin. There are two types of laser treatments performed by dermatologists:

- **Ablative laser resurfacing treatment** uses a laser to remove the epidermis (the outermost skin layer, discussed in more detail earlier in the chapter), while simultaneously heating the deeper tissue. The full healing time is about two to three weeks, and the skin heals with a tighter and firmer tone. Ablative treatment isn't suitable for darker skin since melanin absorbs the laser's energy, and this can lead to scarring.
- **Nonablative laser treatment** doesn't damage the epidermis. It has less risk of complications than ablative treatment, but more treatments are needed to obtain the same results. After a nonablative treatment, the skin is visibly tighter.

Laser treatments are performed using topical anesthesia, although local anesthesia or sedation can be used for certain ablative treatments.

You can also have your neck or other areas laser-treated to firm up the skin.

There are some possible side effects to each procedure, which will usually clear up by themselves as the skin heals. Side effects of ablative laser treatment include bleeding, redness, infection, acne, and crusting. Nonablative treatment can cause some mild pain during the procedure, and redness, blistering, or swelling afterward.

There are home nonablative laser treatment devices available. These machines use lasers that aren't as powerful as those used by dermatologists, and thus it will take longer—generally at least a month—to see results.

Non-Laser Tightening

To stimulate collagen production without a laser, a dermatologist can use radio frequencies or ultrasound. These procedures work in the same way as laser tightening. There are machines available for home use, which will not have the same energy as the machines used by professionals and thus will take longer to show results.

Dermabrasion

Dermabrasion is a form of exfoliation for removing dead skin cells from the epidermal outer layer. Dermabrasion is more intensive than the exfoliating we do at home with scrubbing cleansers and buff puffs. This procedure treats not only fine lines and sun damage but also uneven skin texture, age spots, and acne scars.

Dermabrasion is performed under local anesthesia or sedation by a dermatologist with an instrument called a dermabrader that removes the outer layers of skin. After the procedure, your face will be covered with a moist dressing, and after around three months your face will be completely healed.

Dermaroller/Microneedling

This method is also called collagen induction therapy. During this therapy, your skin is punctured with very small needles to stimulate the healing process, which will trigger the production of new collagen.

Hydration

If your skin isn't properly hydrated, it will lose its plumpness and look aged, tired, and irritated. Your skin locks in moisture with a barrier consisting of fatty acids, cholesterol, and ceramides. Because menopause can result in dry skin, it is important to keep an extra watchful eye on your skin hydration.

You will notice a visible improvement in skin hydration in only a few days if you follow these tips:

- Incorporate essential fatty acids into your diet via foods such as avocado, oily fish, nuts, and vegetable oils, or take a supplement.
- Use a gentle cleanser, but don't overdo it. One cleanse in the morning and one at bedtime is enough. After cleansing, don't dry your face completely. Pat your skin dry to leave it somewhat damp and then apply your moisturizer.
- Drink more water and less coffee and alcohol. Eating water-rich foods will also help increase your total water intake.
- Don't shower or bathe in hot water. Lukewarm is best for your skin.
- Use a hydrating sheet skin mask.

- Avoid salty foods.
- Use your moisturizer every day. You'll get the best results if you use an emollient moisturizer at night.
- Use a humidifier to assist your skin in retaining moisture.
- Help lock moisture in your skin by using skin-care products that contain occlusives (waxes and oils), humectants (glycerin and hyaluronic acid), and emollients (fatty acids, squalene, and ceramides).
- Change your makeup to products containing squalene, hyaluronic acid, or glycerin.

Skin-Tightening Creams

The more elastic the skin is, the more it can bounce back and retain its shape, and the less saggy and loose it will be. For elastic, tight skin, you can consider a cream or lotion that stimulates collagen and prevents sun damage. Such skin-care products will contain these ingredients:

- tretinoin
- retinol
- vitamin E (alpha-tocopherol)
- vitamin B3 (niacinamide)
- vitamin C (L-ascorbic acid)
- hyaluronic acid
- glycolic acid or alpha-hydroxy acid (AHA)
- salicylic acid or beta-hydroxy acid (BHA)
- peptides

Other Cosmetic Procedures

Botox

Botox treatments involve injecting a neurotoxin into a muscle beneath the skin to paralyze it. The newly paralyzed muscle can't contract to cause movement wrinkles, such as frown lines.

Fillers

Unlike PRP injections, dermal filling doesn't rejuvenate the skin or trigger the production of collagen. Dermal fillers are injections of substances that will plump up the skin from underneath. This new plumpness will soften the appearance of wrinkles.

Eyelid Lift

This surgical procedure is called blepharoplasty. In this procedure, a plastic surgeon lifts the eyelids and removes any unwanted fat and sagging skin from the eye area.

Facelift

Also called a rhytidectomy, a facelift is a surgical procedure where the facial skin is pulled tighter and the excess skin is then removed.

One-Stitch Facelift

This procedure, also known as a thread lift, is much less invasive than the classic facelift. A plastic surgeon makes one tiny incision on the hairline at the temple and then passes a single dissolvable stitch through the deep skin layers of the cheeks. When this stitch is tightened, the skin will look instantly tighter.

Neck Lift

There are a number of procedures performed during a full neck lift. Cervicoplasty removes loose, saggy skin (sometimes called neck wattle or turkey neck) from the neck, while platysmaplasty is the realignment and tightening of the neck muscles.

Chemical Peels

A chemical peel has to be done by a specialist to ensure its safety. A chemical is applied to the face that will exfoliate deeply and cause the facial skin to peel off. The new skin that forms will be smoother and have a more even tone, and acne scars and sun damage will be greatly reduced.

There are three classes of chemical peel to choose from, depending on how deeply the chemicals will penetrate the skin:

- **Deep** peels reach the entire middle layer of the skin.
- **Medium** peels reach the outer and upper part of the dermal layer.
- **Superficial** peels exfoliate only the outer layer.

If the phenol or trichloroacetic acid TCA is used for the procedure, anesthesia isn't needed since the chemical solution has anesthetic properties. However, you might be sedated during the procedure to make you more comfortable.

Hair

Menopause can change the way your hair looks and feels. These changes are a natural consequence of hormonal changes. In the following sections, we'll learn more about hair, what changes you might expect during menopause, and what you can do to keep your hair strong, shiny, and plentiful. Let's start by taking a brief look at the structure of hair before diving into the menopausal changes.

Hair isn't just the visible hair shaft but also the part below the skin called the follicle. Hair growth starts in the follicle, which has small blood vessels to nourish the root of the hair. This is why good blood circulation to the scalp is essential for healthy hair growth.

If you pluck out a hair at the root, you'll see a round structure at the base. This is called the bulb and it contains stem cells that will form into hair.

Your scalp contains oil, or sebaceous, glands that border the inner lining of the hair follicle. The oil that the sebaceous glands produce acts as a natural conditioner and moisturizer to your hair shafts. The outer lining of the follicle is attached to a tiny muscle that can contract to give you goosebumps.

The hair shaft itself is made up of an inner, middle, and outer layer, each of which is made from the protein called keratin. The inner and middle layers contain the pigment that gives your hair its color. When you look under a microscope, the outer layer resembles tightly packed roof shingles. Hair conditioners make these "shingles" lie flat and smooth.

If your hair has a circular cross-section, it will fall straight. The flatter the hair's cross-section, the curlier the hair will be. This hair shape also affects how shiny the hair is naturally. Curly hair tends to look duller than straight hair because the oil from the sebaceous glands can't travel as easily down the hair shaft. If your hair shape changes due to the hormonal changes of menopause, you might see a change in shine and oiliness or dryness levels.

Hair Changes

Because estrogen and progesterone affect hair growth and hair follicle health, your hair might grow more slowly and become thinner during menopause. Your scalp's natural oils are also affected by hormones, so menopause can make your hair dull and dry, and your scalp flaky.

You might also find that your hair's texture changes during menopause. Some women's straight hair might become more wavy, while curly hair might straighten. These changes are natural and happen because hormones play a role in the shape of hair follicles so, as hormone levels start fluctuating, the follicles can change their shape accordingly. And, as noted above, it is the shape of your hair follicles that determines the texture of your hair.

The Effects of Chemicals and Styling Tools

You can take handfuls of hair-friendly supplements and use every follicle stimulator on the market, but still won't have healthy hair if you use harsh chemicals and styling tools. Let's take a look at the effects these products and tools have on hair and how you can minimize their damage on the occasions when you do use them:

- **Harsh chemicals** can irritate your scalp, which will lead to itchiness and inflammation. Since scalp health is needed for hair health, chemically induced inflammation will result in hair that's in poor condition. Because hair relaxers, dyes, and perms can strip your hair's natural oils, they can dry out your hair, leading to more tangles and brittle texture.

- **Hair gel, mousse, and hairspray** often contain ingredients that dry out hair and make it brittle. These chemical ingredients can also make your hair frizzy and create flyaways.
- **Styling tools** generally use heat, which can cause damage resulting in split ends, dry hair, and hair that breaks easily. Blow dryers and curling and straightening irons are hot enough to weaken the hair fibers and make them less elastic.

You don't have to stop styling your hair to keep your locks healthy. Stick to salon-grade products and carefully follow the instructions. Keep your use of heat and chemical products to a minimum and use a good conditioner often.

Supplements for Hair Growth

Vitamin B7, also called biotin, plays a part in keratin production. Taking a biotin supplement can help increase the strength and thickness of your hair. If you are vegan, you are at risk of developing a **vitamin B12** deficiency, which can also impact hair growth.

Women are more prone to **iron** deficiency than men. An iron supplement can help remedy hair loss due to deficiency.

Omega-3 fatty acids are necessary for healthy hair follicles. Supplementing with omega-3 fatty acids has the added benefit of increasing the shininess of your hair.

Having low levels of **zinc** can lead to hair loss and slow hair growth.

Taking a supplement can help stimulate your hair growth and reduce hair loss.

Vitamin E is an antioxidant, which means it can protect cells and tissues, including hair follicles, from damage.

If our **vitamin D** levels become low due to lack of sun exposure or being in an office all day, we might experience hair loss. This hair loss can be prevented and treated by taking a vitamin D supplement.

Your body produces keratin from the amino acids in collagen. A **vitamin C** supplement will help synthesize enough collagen to provide the amino acids needed for abundant hair. Vitamin C taken with iron will also make it easier for your body to absorb iron in the intestines.

Most of the supplements for healthy hair can be found in multivitamin supplements that you can take daily. However, don't overdo it! Too high levels of certain vitamins can lead to toxicity and negative side effects. If you are unsure about how much of a supplement you should take, consult your doctor or pharmacist.

Also, if you take a biotin (vitamin B7) supplement, inform your laboratory or doctor when you have blood tests done. This is because biotin can interfere with the testing and lead to inaccurate results.

Pamper Your Scalp

If you have severe hair loss during menopause, you might be able to slow down or reduce the loss by using products containing minoxidil on your scalp. You might also benefit from stimulating your follicles with pulsed red light.

Scalp serums will moisturize your hair while hydrating your scalp. These serums will help stimulate your hair follicles if they contain caffeine and lipids.

Massaging your scalp will not only stimulate hair growth but also help you relax. Stress can contribute to hair loss, so go ahead and treat yourself to a head massage at a beauty salon, use gentle pressure with your own fingertips, or invest in a scalp massage device.

Use rosemary oil as is or combined with jojoba oil to improve your scalp's blood circulation. The better the blood supply, the better and thicker the hair growth.

Massage peppermint oil into your scalp to stimulate oxygen production in your hair follicles. This increased oxygen production can lead to better hair growth.

Condition your scalp with lavender or tea tree oil to open the pores and unclog follicles.

Rub onion juice into your scalp to improve hair growth. The humble onion is rich in sulfur, which stimulates blood flow in the scalp and boosts the production of collagen. Rinsing your hair in onion juice can also help bring the shine back to your hair.

Low-level light therapy uses the energy of laser lights to stimulate blood circulation in the scalp.

Key Takeaways

Because estrogen plays a role in forming and maintaining healthy hair and skin, a lack of estrogen will have visible effects. Menopause can lead to dull or thinning hair, and dry, wrinkly skin. There are various remedies you can try to reverse these effects. Choose the remedy that suits your lifestyle, and don't be scared to experiment.

Chapter 5

Unspoken Fear—Loss of Libido and Reigniting the Spark

*L*ibido is your sex drive and, just like your hormones, it can fluctuate. How much desire you have for sex depends on several factors, including your general health, how secure you feel with your partner, your emotions, and your hormonal state. In this chapter, we'll speak openly about libido, the changes menopause can bring to your sexuality, the effects of low libido on your self-confidence and relationship, and what can be done to bring the spark back into the bedroom.

Picture Clara. After 25 years of marriage, she is still madly in love with her husband. Their sex life had always been sizzling and satisfying—until a few months ago. Paul still charms her with his smile and the way his eyes sparkle when he tells a joke, but she can't muster up any sexual desire. Clara doesn't want to tell Paul that she has lost her libido because she fears that Paul will think he doesn't satisfy her as a lover, or that she doesn't love him anymore. She worries that her lack of desire could ignite arguments that may eventually lead to divorce. So, she tells her husband that she has a headache, is too tired, has a stomach ache, or has to get up early the next day. Clara knows that if she agrees to sex, Paul will notice that she isn't lubricated, and she is worried about how he might interpret that. If only Clara knew that loss of libido and vaginal dryness are normal symptoms of menopause that many other women experience, and that a visit to her doctor could help her out!

An indication that menopause isn't the end of your sex life but the start of a new sexual expression is the spike in sexually transmitted infections (STIs) at age 60 (Ford, 2023). This is more than likely due to the sudden freedom of not having to worry about getting pregnant.

What Determines Libido?

Your brain and biochemistry work together to make you interested in sex. Under certain conditions, your hormones trigger a state of sexual arousal, during which the vagina becomes lubricated and the clitoris enlarges. If you struggle with low libido, these biological processes don't work together to make you desire sexual intimacy.

However, your libido is also influenced by your physical health, psychological state, and medications. Here are some factors that can cause, or exacerbate, the loss of libido:

- smoking
- strains on a relationship
- chronic fatigue
- chronic pain
- chronic illness
- heart disease
- excessive use of alcohol
- negative body image
- hypothyroidism (underactive thyroid)
- previous sexual trauma
- separation, divorce, or death of a partner

- pregnancy
- low self-esteem
- high blood pressure
- anxiety
- anemia
- depression
- some antidepressants
- recreational drugs
- diabetes
- pain or discomfort during sex
- obesity
- stress
- surgical injury to the reproductive organs, blood vessels, or nerves during a hysterectomy
- hormonal fluctuations
- menopause

Signs of a Low Libido

Libido is unique to every individual. There is no medical standard libido level that states a certain amount of sex is too little or too much. However, the following are symptoms of low libido:

- **No, or few, sexual fantasies.** Even the hottest hunk ignites no spark in your imagination.
- **No desire for masturbation.** It is natural to get turned on by a sexy novel or a sizzling movie. If you have low libido, that doesn't happen, and you have no thoughts of taking matters into your own hands.
- **No sexual desire for your partner.** You still love your man but would rather not have sex.

- **Worry about your lack of sexual desire.** This is the stage where low libido starts affecting your everyday life. You worry about your relationship and don't know if your man understands that it really isn't him, it's you—or your hormones, to be more accurate. The worry puts extra strain on you, and this stress lowers your desire for intimacy even more.

Menopausal Changes to the Vagina

Estrogen, the quintessential female hormone, is essential for maintaining the function and health of the female reproductive system. We have already seen that estrogen is produced in the ovaries and plays a role in menstruation and pregnancy. The vagina is also directly dependent on estrogen for its proper function, so when the estrogen supply drops during menopause, the vagina will undergo some changes,. This can have an impact on libido.

When estrogen levels drop, a condition called vaginal atrophy can occur. Vaginal atrophy, also called atrophic vaginitis, is a condition where the vaginal walls become dry, inflamed, and thin due to loss of estrogen. Without proper lubrication and with the vaginal walls inflamed, sex can be at the very least a discomfort, and at most, very painful. It isn't unusual to have spotting after sex since the thinner vaginal walls can tear.

Vaginal atrophy can also affect your urinary system. The following is a list of symptoms you might experience as a result of vaginal atrophy:

- decreased lubrication during sexual arousal
- bleeding (spotting) after sex
- pain or discomfort during sex
- genital itching

- burning sensation in the vulva and vagina (the vulva is the outer part of your genitals)
- vaginal dryness
- vaginal discharge
- tightened and shortened vagina
- urinary incontinence (when you can't hold your pee)
- frequent urination (when you have to plan your trips around bathroom stops)
- burning when you urinate
- recurrent urinary tract infections

Going to the Doctor

Usually, discomfort or pain during sex can be avoided by using a water-based lubricant or a vaginal moisturizer. If that doesn't help, speak to your doctor. There is help available for painful sex and the other symptoms caused by low estrogen.

Your doctor will examine you to find if your vaginal and urinary problems are symptoms of genitourinary syndrome of menopause (GSM). The examination isn't painful. Your doctor will look at your vulva, vagina, and cervix, and feel the inside of your vagina to check for any irregularities of your pelvic organs with two gloved fingers. During the internal exam, your doctor will press down on your abdomen to make it easier for them to feel your uterus, bladder, and ovaries. To test the acid balance of your vagina, your doctor might insert a paper strip or take a sample of your vaginal fluids. You might also have to give a urine sample.

Your doctor might prescribe Addyi, which is a pill that stimulates the brain chemicals responsible for sexual desire, or the Vyleesi injection, which activates areas in the brain that increase libido.

Treating Vaginal Changes

You can take estrogen to relieve the symptoms of menopause, including GSM. Estrogen treatment for GSM can work at low doses and relieve the symptoms directly. Let's take a look at some of the GSM estrogen treatments available.

Topical Estrogen

This is estrogen that is applied directly to the vagina and can be better at relieving vaginal symptoms than taking an estrogen pill. Topical estrogen treatment is available in different forms, and you and your doctor can discuss which treatment will suit you the best. Vaginal tablets and suppositories are inserted directly into the vagina with an applicator. Vaginal estrogen cream is likewise applied to the vagina with an applicator. If you prefer a topical estrogen that you don't have to reapply daily or weekly, you can opt for a vaginal estrogen ring. This soft ring is inserted into the upper part of the vagina and works for about three months.

Other Vaginal Treatments

Your doctor can prescribe lidocaine gel or ointment, which you can apply about 10 minutes before sex to relieve pain and discomfort. You might also consider using vaginal dilators that will counteract menopausal vaginal narrowing by stretching the vaginal muscles. If you are brave regarding needles, you can have the O-shot, which is a plasma injection into the vagina to stimulate blood circulation.

Treating Pelvic Changes: Pelvic Floor Exercises

The muscles of your pelvic floor might become weaker during menopause. This weakening can result in your pelvic organs prolapsing, which means the organs can drop from their proper positions because they aren't fully supported by the muscles anymore. Your bladder, vagina, uterus, rectum, urethra, and small bowel can possibly prolapse. When organs such as the uterus prolapse and push against the bladder or urethra, you won't be able to hold your pee.

Pelvic floor exercises can contribute to the muscle strength of your lower pelvis, and this means that you can improve your bladder and bowel control and treat pelvic organ prolapse without surgery. If you do pelvic floor exercises regularly, not only will you stay dry when you laugh or sneeze, but you'll also have stronger orgasms.

To sense your pelvic floor muscles, imagine you are urinating and have to stop the flow. You will feel some muscles contracting—these are your pelvic floor muscles. Below is how you can exercise them without anyone noticing.

Start by sitting, lying, or standing comfortably, then squeeze your pelvic floor muscles in pulses. Do this 10 times, ensuring you're only contracting your pelvic floor muscles and not your abs, thighs, or glutes. Aim for three sets of 10 repetitions each day. After a week, you can do the same exercise but hold each contraction for two seconds. As this gets easier, you can keep increasing the amount of time you hold the contractions. It's important to carry on doing these exercises regularly; don't make the mistake of stopping when you start noticing results.

Treating Loss of Libido: Aphrodisiacs

An aphrodisiac is a substance that might fire up your love engines, such as chocolate and horny goat weed. In this section, we'll take a look at some common aphrodisiacs to see if they are backed by science. Some substances that are commonly believed to be aphrodisiacs but can't be proven scientifically to influence libido include honey, chasteberry, oysters, and hot chilis.

Maca Root

This Peruvian plant *(Lepidium meyenii)* was the subject of a scientific study that found that maca can improve libido in postmenopausal women who were also taking antidepressants (Dording et al., 2015). Maca might also act as an aphrodisiac by helping to balance estrogen levels in perimenopausal women and relieving hot flashes and night sweats in menopausal women. Not having to deal with hot flashes clears the way for hot action in the bedroom!

Because maca root can influence hormones, it is better to use a different libido treatment if you are being treated for estrogen-related breast or uterine cancer or have any thyroid problems.

Horny Goat Weed

The name itself is a clue that this plant (*Epimendium grandiflorum*) has a reputation for spicing up the libido. Horny goat weed, known in traditional Chinese medicine as *yin yang huo*, contains plant estrogens and substances that enhance blood circulation (*Horny Goat Weed*, n.d.). If you are pregnant, avoid horny goat weed because it might cause harm to your fetus.

Red Ginseng

A study has shown that red ginseng can boost libido in menopausal women. The scientists discovered that red ginseng affects the clitoral muscle and the muscle in the vagina (Oh et al., 2010). If you plan to try red ginseng to enhance your libido, speak to your doctor or pharmacist first if you are undergoing treatment for an estrogen-sensitive cancer or are using blood thinners.

Fenugreek

Fenugreek (*Trigonella foenum-graecum*) is well-known in Ayurvedic medicine as a treatment for low libido, and one study has found that fenugreek seeds have the same effect as estrogen (Sreeja et al., 2010). It might also increase breast size (Yadav & Baquer, 2013).

Like all other remedies and supplements that have the same effect as estrogen, fenugreek is unsuitable for women who are being treated for estrogen-sensitive cancers.

Chocolate

Eating chocolate isn't just a sensual sweet melting on your tongue, it is also a chemical mood enhancer. It boosts serotonin, which is the happiness hormone. The darker the chocolate, the richer it is in cacao, and the happier you might feel. The sensuality and serotonin boost of chocolate makes it the aphrodisiac of choice for sweet-toothed romantics.

Saffron

This is the most expensive spice and is made from the flower of *Crocus sativus*. Spending a small fortune on a spice might be worth it, judging by a study that found women who used saffron experienced more sexual arousal and lubrication than women who didn't consume the spice (Kashani et al., 2012).

Ashwagandha

This Ayurvedic remedy might lower stress hormones and help regulate testosterone, which improves libido in both sexes. An ingredient in ashwagandha (*Withania somnifera)* called withanolide can help induce quality sleep, which can also contribute to an increased desire for sex.

Shatavari

The name of this Ayurvedic remedy hints at its use; *shatavari* means "she who has 100 husbands"! Although it is doubtful whether shatavari (*Asparagus racemosus*) can give you the stamina to deal with the 100 loads of laundry, 100 missing briefcases, or 100 other issues that 100 husbands might bring, it might just perk up your sex drive enough to at least fantasize about 100 husbands.

Shatavari stimulates blood flow to the genitals, which makes sex more pleasurable and can help improve vaginal lubrication. Not only do the plant estrogens in shatavari help turn your thoughts toward sex, they also help reduce vaginal inflammation and balance hormones.

Treating Loss of Libido

Reducing Stress

It isn't always possible to reduce stressful circumstances, but you may be able to de-stress before bed. In this section, we'll look at some techniques that can help restore inner calm and lower the stress hormones that interfere with libido.

Breathing

Deep breathing exercises can benefit your sex drive in two ways. Firstly, you'll be more relaxed, and your sexual response won't have to compete with stress hormones. Secondly, your blood will be more oxygenated, which can enhance your libido.

You might have heard of the combination of Buddhist breathing, yoga, and meditation techniques called tantra. Tantric exercises focus on sexual energy and can improve libido by enhancing the flow of oxygenated blood throughout the entire body. Let's try a tantric breathing exercise to relax you and help you to get more in touch with your senses.

Take a slow, deep breath. While you are inhaling, feel how the breath fills you from your sexual organs to the top of your head. During your slow exhalation, pay attention to your body. Notice subtle changes in your senses from the beginning of the exhale to when your lungs are empty. Repeat this breathing meditation as many times as you're comfortable. You can also do this with a partner and try to sync your breathing.

Meditation

Meditation can make you more aware of your body and put you in touch with sensations you've seldom paid attention to before. This can not only revitalize your sex drive but also make sex feel new and more pleasurable.

Yoga

There are some yoga poses that stimulate blood flow to the genital region. Not only can these poses help you to relax deeply, but they may also improve your sexual sensation and libido. Here are two yoga poses that improve pelvic blood flow:

- The Queen of the Frogs
  - This pose is also known as *Malasana*. To start, stand up straight with your feet hip-width apart. Put your hands together in front of your chest as if you were praying. Keep your hands in this position and lower your glutes until you are in a deep squat.
  - While you are in the deep squat position, touch your inner thighs lightly with your elbows and keep your shoulders pulled back so that your back is straight. Hold this position while you breathe deeply five times, then return to the starting position.
  - If you find this position too difficult, you can modify it. Instead of sinking into a deep squat, lower your glutes only as far down as you find comfortable. Even if you lower yourself only a few inches and gradually work up to more, you'll enjoy improved pelvic blood circulation.
- The Cobra

- The cobra pose, also known as *Bhujangasana*, can not only improve pelvic blood circulation and sexual sensitivity but also strengthen your hips and core and increase your spinal mobility.
- Start the cobra by lying face down on a rug, towel, or yoga mat. Put your palms next to your shoulders and inhale slowly. Slowly and gently lift only your upper body. Don't hunch your shoulders up toward your ears. When your upper body is fully raised off the floor, you can either look up to the ceiling if you don't have neck problems, or you can look straight ahead.
- Hold this pose for 10 counts. Then, while exhaling slowly, lower your upper body back down. You can do five cobra poses at a time and increase the amount gradually until you can do 10 in a session.

Tai Chi

Tai chi is a gentle but effective form of exercise that incorporates graceful, flowing movements to release tension, improve mobility and muscle tone, and restore energy. The movements help you become more aware of your body, and this will help you reconnect with your sexuality and sensual experience.

Dancing

Going dancing can help improve your blood circulation and increase your blood oxygen levels, which can make you feel more alive, energetic, and sexy. It's a fun way to de-stress while you spend time away from the house with your partner.

Cognitive Behavioral Therapy

Cognitive behavioral therapy (CBT) is a psychological method that can help with issues such as depression and loss of libido. It identifies and addresses negative thought patterns as well as problems in a relationship that can reduce your desire for intimacy. CBT can help you communicate with your partner about the menopausal changes you are going through, what concerns you have about your libido, and what you can do to reignite the spark.

Libido Killers to Try to Avoid

Stress

Having a particularly stressful day, or being under stress for a long time, isn't just exhausting and distracting but can physically lower your libido. When you are under stress, your body gets flooded with the stress-response hormones cortisol and adrenaline. These stress hormones affect your overall hormonal balance and can also narrow your arteries, including those that carry blood to your genitals, resulting in low sexual response.

Many of us enjoy having a leisurely bubble bath by candlelight to relax and initiate a sensual evening. However, bear in mind that bubble baths can result in the development of vaginitis, such as yeast infections. The vagina has an acidic pH balance (pH is a scale of how acidic or alkaline something is), which is necessary for the protective micro-organisms to flourish. Bubble baths can upset this pH balance, which may lead to symptoms such as vaginal itching, infection, and dryness. Bubble bath products can contain substances such as artificial fragrances and dye that can negatively affect the friendly vaginal bacteria, leading to conditions such as thrush, inflammation, and bacterial vaginosis. Glitter in bath bombs can scratch the vaginal lining, glycerin breaks down into sugar which provides a feast for yeast, and phthalates and parabens can disrupt your hormones.

If you are prone to vaginal infections, it is therefore advisable to stay out of bubble baths.

Alcohol

A glass of wine before intimacy can help lower your inhibitions and make you feel seductive. Alcohol might also help you relax, and there is something sensual about sipping pink champagne or gazing into your lover's eyes over a glass of red wine. However, overdoing it results in loss of libido, nausea, and hangovers, which are not sexy.

Licorice Root

Licorice contains a substance called glycyrrhizin, which can lower libido. Glycyrrhizin can drop your potassium levels, cause you to retain fluid, throw your hormones off balance, and elevate your blood pressure. High doses can even lead to fatigue, muscle weakness, and heart issues. Having a little bit of licorice now and then is fine, but be aware that overdoing it can cause you to lose interest in the bedroom.

Depression

Being depressed can alter your body chemistry, and this can interfere with your interest in sex. Some antidepressants can also cause your libido to dry up. Above all, if you have depression, you may simply not be in the mood for sex. There is help, though. Your doctor can prescribe an antidepressant that won't interfere with your body's sexual response, and this can improve your mood overall.

Mint

Mint products contain menthol, which can lower testosterone. We tend to associate testosterone only with the male sex drive, but women also need small amounts of testosterone to help maintain libido. Researchers found that spearmint tea (*Mentha spicata*) can lower testosterone levels in women (Grant, 2010).

Sleep Deprivation

Sleepless nights due to night sweats, insomnia, or late-night TV can leave your body starved of sleep. This can cause you to fall asleep the moment your head hits the pillow, even though you may be in the mood for sex. Your body needs sleep to survive, and if your brain has to choose between essential sleep or sex, it won't choose sex. A lack of sleep can also raise your cortisol levels, which will suppress your libido.

Low Self-Esteem

Being sweaty from hot flashes, having dry skin, hair thinning, or weight gain are all potential side effects of losing estrogen during menopause. You know that these are natural changes and that your body needs time to adjust to the lower estrogen levels, but these changes can still affect your self-esteem. If you feel uncomfortable in your body or unattractive, you might not want physical intimacy.

Painful or Uncomfortable Sex

Estrogen plays a part in maintaining our vaginal health. When estrogen levels fall, we may have symptoms such as vaginal dryness and itchiness and thinning vaginal walls. This can lead to sex being uncomfortable or downright painful, and there might be some light bleeding afterward. Being in pain doesn't go well with a romantic evening. Fortunately, your doctor can prescribe an estrogen cream that you can apply topically to your vagina, or other products that can help restore your vaginal health.

Relationship Issues

Anything that affects your relationship can also affect your desire for sex. Having an argument, communication problems, resenting something your partner has said or done, or financial difficulties can make you less likely to want to feel physically close to your partner.

Reigniting the Spark

Taking care of your body and getting medical and therapeutical help, if needed, will go a long way toward raising your libido. Here are some more tips on how to bring the passion back in your relationship:

- Start simply by holding hands and making more eye contact.
- Have date nights, or other designated times where it's only the two of you doing something fun.
- Show affection physically by hugging, giving a back massage, or touching your partner's arm when you speak. Cuddle up next to each other in front of the TV, play footsie under the

kitchen table, and snuggle together in bed. All of these actions will help rekindle emotional intimacy, which may lead to the desire for sex.

- Explore different aspects of sexuality. Visit a sex shop or browse the internet for various sex aids. Try something different that makes you feel a little bit naughty, such as wearing sexy lingerie, buying a lubricant, or trying a vibrator.
- Build sexual tension through sharing sexual fantasies, watching a sexy movie together, spending more time on foreplay, or sharing a romantic light dinner before getting physically intimate.
- Stop blaming each other, or yourself, for the lack of spark in the bedroom. Loss of libido can happen to any couple for various reasons. Move past the blame and talk to each other about what you can do to rekindle the flame.
- Visit your doctor to treat physical issues that steal your sex drive. Symptoms such as vaginal dryness, uncomfortable or painful intercourse, and lack of interest in sex can be medically treated.

Break the Taboo

For many women, talking about sex is something that makes them feel uncomfortable. Mentioning menopause may be equally difficult. Because of this, many women suffer in silence and wouldn't dream of telling their doctor, therapist, or pharmacist that they are experiencing loss of libido, discomfort during sex, or vaginal dryness.

Rest assured that your health professional is trained to deal with issues regarding menopause and sexuality. They have undergone years of professional training to help you and have heard it all—and worse—before. They won't judge you, laugh at you, or think there is something wrong with you. Also, people in health professions are required by their licensing boards to be discreet.

Key Takeaways

Menopause can affect hormones in such a way that your sex drive takes a back seat. Fortunately, there are treatments available for the various menopausal causes of low libido. Remember that your health professional is trained to help you without judgment, and the treatments they can prescribe may change your life, libido, and relationship for the better.

If you are one of the lucky women who has a fully intact libido, you might be tempted to celebrate your freedom from the risk of pregnancy with sexy adventures. You might feel like a teenager again, ready to experiment and go wild! You might even give a patrol cop a raised eyebrow if he shines his flashlight into the parked cars in "lovers' lane" only to see two "old folks" having a bit of naughty fun. What's he going to do, call your parents and have you grounded? Have fun and explore your post-period sexuality, but use a condom. You might not have to worry about changing nappies in nine months, but an STI can cramp your style. With all the flavored, colored, and textured condoms available, you can be safe *and* sexy.

In the next chapter, we'll discuss the emotional roller coaster of mood swings and how to handle them.

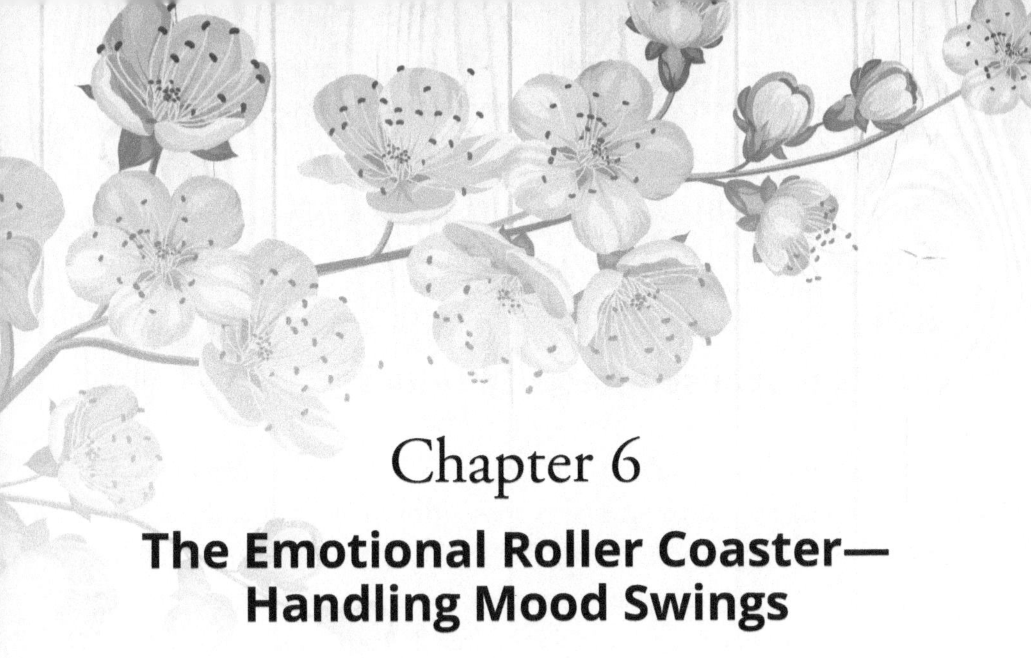

Chapter 6

The Emotional Roller Coaster— Handling Mood Swings

*I*magine riding a roller coaster. Your heart may race at the thought of the scary climbs followed by the fast drop and the terrifying speed of the ride while being in a small car high above the ground. For many menopausal women, their emotions are on a roller coaster all day. It can be terrifying to experience a sudden fall into deep, unexplained sadness followed by a sense of trepidation, topped off by a few minutes of irritation. In this chapter, we'll explore the emotional side of the menopause journey. Let's start by discovering what emotions are and how they originate in the brain.

The Brain's Role in Emotions

The part of your brain responsible for emotions is called the limbic system. The limbic system consists of four different structures, and these work together to make you feel emotions such as love, anger, fear, and happiness. When your brain generates an emotion, it sends a message to the hypothalamus to signal the relevant glands that it is time to release a certain hormone. For example, if you are afraid, your brain tells your adrenal glands to release adrenalin. If you feel love, your brain causes the release of hormones such as oxytocin, vasopressin, and dopamine.

How Menopause Affects Emotions

Because your brain causes your emotions to be experienced through the effects of hormones, it makes sense that when your hormones are unbalanced, your emotions will be as well. As we saw in a previous chapter, during menopause the production of progesterone and estrogen shifts from your ovaries to your adrenal glands, and this change, as well as the lower hormonal levels, can make some women experience emotional changes.

The following emotional effects can be traced to hormonal changes during menopause:

- mood swings
- irritability
- anxiety
- depression
- difficulty focusing
- trouble with recall
- low self-esteem
- lower self-confidence
- anger
- sadness
- tearfulness

These symptoms may come and go. If your emotions are affected by hormonal changes, you might find yourself angry one minute and sad the next. Fortunately, there are ways you can help tame hormonal moods.

How You Can Stabilize Your Moods

After a few months or years, depending on your unique biochemistry, your body will get used to the change in estrogen levels and adjust accordingly. If you've been struggling with emotional changes during the transition period, you'll find your emotions more stable when your body has adjusted. Unfortunately, there isn't a way to predict how long that will take. In the meantime, there are several things you can do to help keep your moods from running amok.

Exercise

One of the hormones that is responsible for making you feel the emotion of happiness is serotonin. When you exercise, your body's production of serotonin is stimulated. Exercise can also help relieve some stress, which will decrease the levels of the stress hormone cortisol. Since cortisol also plays a part in weight gain, you'll not only feel happier but also lose weight more easily if you stick to a regular exercise routine.

Diet

Eating foods that are rich in phytoestrogens (plant estrogens) can give your body enough of an estrogen boost to relieve some of the symptoms of menopause. You might see an improvement in hot flashes, libido, sleep, and mood if you add certain foods to your plate.

Some of the phytoestrogen-rich foods that can help iron out your mood swings are soy, grapes, berries, flaxseeds, plums, and chickpeas. The menopausal drop in estrogen can also lead to a loss of muscle mass, so remember to add more protein to your diet to help maintain your muscles.

There are some foods that can also influence your mood. When you eat food that gets digested quickly, such as white bread, your blood sugar levels can fluctuate. Not only can this lead to a greater possibility of type 2 diabetes and heart disease, it can also leave you feeling tired and cranky. To have a more gradual increase in your blood sugar levels, choose foods that are digested more slowly (also referred to as having a low glycemic index or GI), such as whole grains.

Here are some tips to help you choose foods with a low GI:

- Fatty and acidic foods are generally low GI.
- The more processed the food, the more likely it is to have a high GI.
- Whole grains have a lower GI than processed grains because the finer the grains, the faster they are digested.
- Fruits have a lower GI before they fully ripen. Ripe fruits and vegetables are high-GI foods.
- Foods that are high in fiber take longer to digest, meaning that they are blood sugar friendly and low GI.
- Add more nuts to your diet, since they are packed with good fats and high fiber. However, you should pay attention to your body's response to nuts, and cut down if you have diarrhea or constipation.

Sleep

Menopause can cause some women to have insomnia. If you can't sleep, exhaustion will build up until it interferes with your moods. Often, night sweats and hot flashes are to blame for interrupting your sleep. If you have hot flashes, your brain undergoes certain biochemical changes that will trigger a hot flash. When these changes occur in the brain, it can cause you to wake up just in time to have a hot flash.

Having lower estrogen and progesterone can contribute to sleep apnea and other sleep disorders. Sleep apnea is a condition where people repeatedly stop and start breathing in their sleep. This happens when either the throat muscles relax so much that they block the airflow, or the brain doesn't regulate the breathing muscles correctly. Sleep apnea prevents a good night's sleep, and the resulting fatigue can interfere with mood the next day.

If you suspect you might have sleep apnea, speak to your doctor about treatment. The symptoms of sleep apnea are

- being sleepy during the day
- irritability
- loud snoring
- waking up with a headache
- waking up with a dry mouth
- if you share your bed, your partner noticing that you gasp for breath or stop breathing while you sleep

Relaxation

When you relax, your levels of cortisol and adrenaline fall, leading to more balanced hormones. The more your hormones are balanced, the smoother your moods should be. You can experiment with various relaxation techniques to find the method that is best for you. Some relaxation methods you might want to try are as follows:

- **Autonomous sensory meridian response (ASMR).** Have you ever had tingles when the hairdresser styles your hair or when someone whispers in your ear? This is ASMR, and there are thousands of YouTube videos available with various sounds and scenarios to relax you with tingles.

- **Binaural beats.** These are beats created by your brain when you listen to a different tone in each ear. Your brain will make you hear a third tone. Your brainwaves can sync up to this third beat to create various effects, including becoming more relaxed or helping you sleep. You can find binaural beats online, and all you need to enjoy their relaxing effect is a pair of earbuds or headphones.

- **Guided meditation.** You can find thousands of guided meditations online to help you relax or fall asleep more easily. In a guided meditation session, you listen to someone leading you along the relaxation process, usually by telling you to progressively relax your muscles. This is often followed by a guided visualization accompanied by soothing music.

- **Breathing techniques.** The yoga technique called pranayama is all about breath control. Some pranayama methods can help you relax and fall asleep. Among the most popular pranayama methods is 4–7–8 breathing, so-called because you slowly inhale for four seconds, after which you hold your breath for seven seconds, then follow this with a slow exhale for eight seconds.

- **Tai chi.** This form of exercise involves flowing, graceful, slow movements that tone the muscles while relaxing the mind. You can find instructional videos online or join a class with a qualified, experienced instructor.

- **Yoga.** Yoga is the umbrella term for diverse types of movements, poses, and breathing techniques. For relaxation and calming emotions, restorative yoga and yin yoga are the most suitable forms. Both forms are beginner friendly and don't involve twisting yourself into poses that make you feel like a human pretzel. Restorative yoga helps you cleanse your mind of the stresses of the day, while yin yoga includes seated postures to help you relax and balance your emotions.

Cognitive Behavioral Therapy

This type of therapy focuses on identifying and addressing behavioral patterns. CBT can help you with menopausal mood disorders such as depression and anxiety. Any qualified mental health professional will be able to answer the questions you may have regarding this form of therapy.

HRT

Unless you have severe depression that needs to be treated with antidepressant therapy, HRT can help even out your moods. HRT can also help with symptoms that indirectly affect your moods, such as insomnia, weight gain, and hot flashes.

Miscellaneous Tips

Here are some more tips on how you can take control of your emotions during menopause:

- **Get creative.** Take an art or craft course, or do something creative at home where you can express your feelings visibly through drawing, sculpting, scrapbooking, knitting, or other crafts.
- **Stay connected.** If you have friends or family nearby, go and visit or invite them over for a cup of coffee. Use the internet and social media to make new friends and stay in contact with family, friends, and acquaintances who live far away. Having a social network for emotional support can work wonders for improving mood.

- **Join a club.** It can be easier to commit to an exercise routine if you exercise in a group, so why not join a sports club? There are clubs and groups for almost every interest. If you join, you can do or talk about something you enjoy with like-minded people. For women who might struggle with feelings of loneliness or boredom during menopause, a club can help relieve those feelings. If you can't find a club to match your interests, you could take the initiative and start one yourself!

- **Keep a journal.** Your journal is always there to listen to your feelings, fears, and triumphs. Going through menopause can be a lonely time if you feel your family and friends don't understand how it is impacting you. If you don't have someone with whom you can talk about your moods and other menopause symptoms, write your experiences down in a trusty journal instead.

- **Try a supplement**. There are natural remedies available that can help to stabilize your moods directly or indirectly by reducing uncomfortable symptoms. These remedies include
  - ginseng to boost mood and increase energy
  - black cohosh to reduce hot flashes
  - red clover to supply phytoestrogens
  - St. John's wort, especially in combination with black cohosh, to help ease mild depression and reduce mood swings

- **Make note.** Be aware of what you eat or drink before you experience mood swings. There might be something in your diet that triggers mood swings, such as coffee, tea, energy drinks, or sugary and spicy food.

Social Media Warning

If you use social media or an online group or club to share your experiences, get or give support, or make new friends, be careful. A phenomenon called catfishing is a danger that can easily ensnare you if you don't know the warning signs. A catfish is someone who pretends to be in love with you online to extort money from you. They build a relationship with you until you are hooked, and then, when it is time to meet in person, they have some financial crisis that prevents them from traveling to you. Often, they use the excuses that they are working in a foreign country and are not allowed to leave unless they pay their contractors a large amount of money, that they are required to pay a substantial sum to officials, or even that they have been kidnapped and you must help pay the ransom!

In most cases, the catfish will tell you that they are financially very well-off but can't access their money at the moment, or that they are waiting for a large settlement or inheritance to be paid out. A catfish may ask you to give them the traveling costs to come visit you, or other sums that will enable the two of you to start a life together. After you've paid the money into their account, you can bet that they'll come up with a new excuse as to why they can't come and see you in the flesh.

A catfish will often have an accent that doesn't match their backstory, or they will have excuses why you can't phone them whenever you want. They also won't have video conversations (FaceTime) with you, and the photos they send you will be of someone else. Do a Google image search of any photos someone sends you, and insist on a video call before considering an online romance.

Key Takeaways

Not all menopausal women will experience alterations in mood, but for those who do, there are ways to help reduce the effects of estrogen loss on the brain's emotional centers. From pharmaceuticals to natural remedies and self-care, there is help available to make your menopausal journey less of an emotional roller coaster.

In the next chapter, we'll stay with the effects of changing estrogen levels on the brain and discover why and how your memory is sometimes less sharp during menopause.

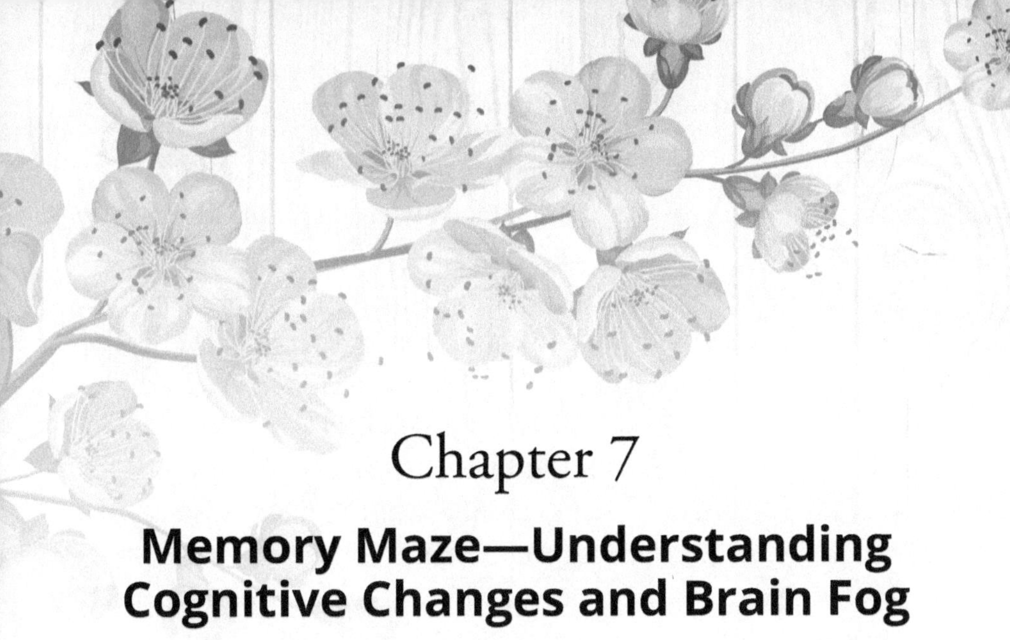

Chapter 7

Memory Maze—Understanding Cognitive Changes and Brain Fog

Imagine Heather, a 60-year-old tax accountant. She was top of her class from first grade to college, and her hobbies include learning new languages and reading everything she can find about organic chemistry. Heather is brilliant, with a sharp wit and kindness that make her eyes sparkle.

Heather's periods stopped six years ago. Her hot flashes are becoming less severe, but her brain fog seems to be getting worse. During a recent meeting with a client, Heather suddenly forgot the word for tax. One moment she was explaining a new regulation regarding tax breaks to an important corporate client, and the next moment she just stood there, trying to find the word for the money owed to the government. Heather had experienced a few memory lapses before, where she couldn't remember where she put her coffee, what her phone number was, or why she had opened the fridge. But not remembering a word she used several times each day caused her not only embarrassment but also intense worry.

The first thing Heather did when she got back from the meeting was look up dementia and Alzheimer's disease. She cried as she made an appointment with her doctor, convinced that life as she knew it was over.

Her doctor sent her for blood tests and gave her a questionnaire. When he called her with the results a few days later, he asked her to see him to discuss her treatment. Heather was surprised when she was prescribed HRT and given a list of suggested dietary supplements and lifestyle changes. Her doctor said that her memory was fine but her recall wasn't as sharp as it used to be. She wasn't in the early stages of a neurological disorder; she was menopausal.

In this chapter, we're exploring why and how menopause affects memory, and what you can do to reclaim your brain. Let's start by investigating memory and recall.

Memory and Recall

To understand the difference between memory and recall, picture your mind as a vast warehouse filled with near-endless filing cabinets. Everything that ever happens to you, every word you read, every sound you hear, every sight you see, every experience, dream, fantasy, and interaction, is neatly put in a file, labeled, and stored in one of the millions of filing cabinets. The filing, organizing, and storing of your perceptions, thoughts, and experiences are your memories.

Recall is telling your mind's filing clerk to retrieve a specific file. For example, if you are at the store and wondering if you should buy a can of soup, your virtual filing clerk runs to the file labeled "soup" and speed-reads the file to get to the memory of your hubby asking you to pick him up a can of tomato soup. This retrieval and accessing of memories is recall.

How Menopause Affects Cognition

Your nervous system, including the brain, consists of nerve cells. When estrogen levels drop from perimenopause onward, the nerve cells are affected and undergo several changes. The nerve cells can change shape and number. They change the way they use glucose for energy, and can start accumulating abnormal proteins. There can be changes in the connections nerve cells form, and the brain structure can also change.

A symptom of menopausal brain changes is hot flashes, which occur when the area of the brain responsible for temperature regulation doesn't get enough estrogen to activate properly. A lack of estrogen can also cause insomnia because the brainstem in charge of the sleep and wake cycle doesn't get activated in the right way. Memory and mood are affected when estrogen levels fall and rise in the brain's memory and emotional areas. This hormonal instability causes mood swings and forgetfulness.

While your body is still adapting to the changes in estrogen levels, your brain's gray matter will decline. Fortunately, your body will adapt and your gray matter will return to normal. You can either wait out the process or take HRT to treat these brain changes.

During the time when your body is still learning how to deal with fluctuating and declining estrogen levels, you may experience cognitive symptoms that affect your speech. These symptoms include a decline in verbal processing speed, delayed verbal memory, and reduced verbal learning. You may forget words, take longer to understand what someone is saying, or struggle to remember what you've heard. These symptoms are natural and not signs of dementia. All of these symptoms will go away after menopause (how long after menopause depends on the individual), and your brain will return to normal.

Your hot flashes and night sweats can also exacerbate your memory problems by decreasing blood flow. After you have a hot episode, your cortisol levels can remain high for a further 20 minutes, and this can negatively affect your memory.

Nootropics

Nootropics are also called brain boosters or smart drugs. They are substances that help you remember and concentrate better and feel more focused, motivated, and creative. People who take nootropics for better brain performance are called neurohackers. In this section, we'll take a look at some nootropics that can help your brain function better during your menopause journey. Nootropic dosages vary according to the manufacturer. If you have any questions about a nootropic, speak to your pharmacist, nutritionist, or doctor before trying a product.

Caffeine

If you enjoy a cup of coffee in the morning to clear your mind, you are a neurohacker. A cup of coffee can chase the brain fog away by blocking a substance called adenosine in your brain. This will help you feel more alert and better able to focus on a task. Caffeine is found in supplement form, or in guarana, coffee beans, tea, cocoa, and kola nuts. Most energy drinks contain caffeine.

The more caffeine you take in during the day, the more likely you are to experience side effects such as jitteriness, anxiety, insomnia, headaches, rapid heartbeat, and dizziness. If you aren't used to caffeine, start with a low dose and gradually increase your caffeine intake.

Aniracetam

This nootropic was patented in 1978 and is available as a supplement in the US and as a prescription drug in the EU. Aniracetam helps the brain repair damaged cell membranes and sharpens focus and concentration. It is also used by neurohackers to increase brain energy, which leads to better recall and memory.

Aniracetam has several other effects on the brain. When combined with caffeine, it makes it easier to study or work for long sessions. It can also enhance the pleasure of listening to music, make it easier to articulate your thoughts, and make colors look more vibrant.

Taking more than the manufacturer's recommended dosage can cause you to experience nausea, anxiety, and fatigue. If you take aniracetam without also taking choline supplements, you may have headaches.

Holy Basil

Holy basil, also called tulsi, helps to increase your reward hormone (dopamine) and happiness hormone (serotonin) while reducing cortisol (the stress hormone), which enables you to relax and feel good. Holy basil can protect the brain against toxins and make your memory and thinking sharper.

If you have diabetes, it is safer to avoid holy basil except in small amounts as used in food preparation. This is because holy basil can cause a sharp drop in blood sugar.

People who are sensitive to a certain compound found in holy basil called eugenol may experience side effects such as diarrhea and a fast heart rate.

Ginkgo Biloba

This extract from the ginkgo tree can increase blood flow in the brain, which makes more oxygen and glucose available to the brain cells to boost recall, memory, and learning. Combined with its effects as a mood booster and stress reliever, ginkgo biloba is a favorite of many neurohackers. However, to experience the full benefits of ginkgo biloba, it is recommended that you use it continuously for several weeks (Tomen, 2023a).

Ginkgo biloba isn't for everyone. It can interact negatively with some medications, which is why ginkgo biloba should be avoided by people who are taking antidepressants, blood thinners, herbs containing coumarin (ask your pharmacist if you are taking herbal remedies), St. John's wort, seizure medication, insulin, or melatonin.

NADH

NADH, also called coenzyme 1, can help provide your brain cells with more energy and stimulate the release of neurotransmitters that play a role in memory, recall, cognition, mood, and learning. It also increases the blood flow to the brain and protects your brain cells from damage. Because NADH occurs naturally in every cell in your body, taking it in supplement form is very unlikely to have any negative side effects.

Coenzyme Q-10

The "batteries" of every cell in your body are little organelles called mitochondria. The mitochondria take substances and convert them into energy. Your brain uses so much energy that the greatest concentration of mitochondria in your body is in your brain cells. Without coenzyme Q-10, your mitochondria can't produce energy.

When you take a coenzyme Q-10 supplement, you provide your brain with more energy, which helps you think more clearly and quickly. As an added benefit, coenzyme Q-10 can also help reduce fatigue.

If you have low blood pressure, speak to your doctor or pharmacist before trying coenzyme Q-10 since it may cause your blood pressure to drop even lower. Side effects from coenzyme Q-10 are rare but may include diarrhea, skin rash, and nausea.

Huperzine-A

Huperzine-A is sourced from the Chinese club moss plant. It enhances brain function by improving short-term memory and helping mitochondria to function at their best. Because it is also an antioxidant, it protects the brain against damage and helps brain cells live longer.

If you have asthma, emphysema, or any blockages in your urinary tract, taking Huperzine-A can make your symptoms worse. It is also an unsuitable supplement for people with epilepsy and heart disease.

Tyrosine

Taking a tyrosine nootropic supplement can help you reduce anxiety, think more clearly, and improve your mood. These effects occur because your brain converts tyrosine into L-dopa, which is then further converted into dopamine. The increased dopamine can help you concentrate better.

Because tyrosine stimulates certain areas of the brain's prefrontal cortex, it helps boost thinking and creativity. Avoid thyrosine supplements if you use thyroid medication, MAO inhibitors, or are prone to migraines.

Yoga

At first glance, it might seem odd to recommend yoga poses and breathing methods to restore memory and cognition, but a study has shown that yoga can affect the brain. The study focused on senior citizens who didn't have dementia and tested the effects of six months of yoga meditation, breathing, and poses. It was found that the study volunteers saw improvements in attention span, verbal and visual memory, and processing speed (Brenes et al., 2019).

Herbal Remedies to Boost Memory

Another weapon in your fight against menopausal memory issues is the traditional ancient natural medicine practice Ayurveda. Many Ayurvedic remedies are available as dietary supplements, so if you don't like measuring out or ingesting dried herbs, you can opt for a capsule or tablet instead. Let's take a look at some Ayurvedic and other herbal remedies you can use to boost your memory during, and after, menopause.

Rosemary

Adding rosemary (*Rosmarinus officinalis*) to your food, or enjoying it in your tea to enhance the flavor, can help your memory and speed up your thinking. You can also use rosemary as an essential oil to boost your memory and thinking processes.

A study has shown that diffused rosemary aroma (inhaling rosemary essential oil) helped volunteers think more accurately and faster (Moss & Oliver, 2012). Another study found that taking a low dose of rosemary powder resulted in faster memory processing (Pengelly et al., 2012).

If you take rosemary as a supplement, remember that less is more regarding dosage. Taking 4–6 g per day will benefit your memory, but more than that can lead to side effects such as muscle spasms and vomiting.

Ingesting large amounts of rosemary can lead to side effects such as vomiting, seizures, fluid buildup in the lungs, and intestinal irritation. Excessive amounts of rosemary can stimulate menstruation and may cause a miscarriage in pregnant women.

Ginseng

The memory-enhancing effect of ginseng (*Panax ginseng*) is due to its active components called ginsengosides. Not only can ginsenosides give the immune system a boost, but they can also help increase neuroplasticity. Neuroplasticity is your brain's ability to make new connections, which is how the brain remembers and learns. Because ginseng also improves blood flow to the brain, the brain receives more oxygen, and this helps improve the ability to concentrate.

Take ginseng supplements with food to make it easier for your body to absorb the ginsenosides. Stick to the dosage recommended on the product label to avoid side effects such as headaches and an upset stomach.

If you are taking any of these medications, speak to your doctor or pharmacist first before trying ginseng: medication to treat diabetes, blood pressure, or heart conditions, or blood thinners.

To avoid adverse effects such as insomnia and nausea, don't take more ginseng than the FDA's recommended 4 g daily (Modi & Modi, 2022).

Gotu Kola

Gotu kola (*Centella asiatica*) has several active ingredients that boost cognition and improve mood. One study showed that gotu kola improved the memory and mood of the study volunteers (Wattanathorn et al., 2008).

It is generally safe to take gotu kola supplements, but taking them long term, especially at high doses (the appropriate dosage varies according to the manufacturers and will be printed on the label or package insert), can increase the risk of experiencing side effects. The potential side effects of gotu kola include nausea, drowsiness, headache, and dizziness.

Because gotu kola can have negative interactions with certain medications, it is safer to speak to your doctor or pharmacist if you plan to take gotu kola while also using medications that can affect the liver, or medications to treat diabetes, cholesterol, water retention, anxiety, or insomnia.

Bacopa

Bacopa (*Bacopa monnieri*), also known as *brahmi*, has a long Ayurvedic tradition of enhancing cognition, memory, and learning.

Bacopa supplements come with various recommended doses, and the doses are generally safe when they are less than 600 mg per day. However, there haven't been any studies to determine its long-term safety. So, err on the side of caution and don't take bacopa for more than 12 weeks continuously (*Bacopa—Uses, Side Effects, and More*, n.d.).

The potential side effects of bacopa include nausea, stomach cramps, and dry mouth. Due to negative interactions, bacopa isn't a suitable supplement if you have a heart condition, a stomach ulcer, a urinary or gastrointestinal tract blockage, a lung condition, or a thyroid disorder.

Speak to your pharmacist or doctor before taking bacopa if you are taking any prescription medication.

Sweet Basil

Sweet basil (*Ocimum basilicum*) can be used as an essential oil to enhance focus and memory while reducing stress and fatigue. To enhance your brain power, mix a drop of sweet basil oil with half a teaspoon of castor oil and massage the mixture into your temples (Banbury, n.d.).

The scent of essential oil helps strengthen and stimulate memory because the area of the brain that processes scent and the area responsible for memory are very close together.

If you plan on using basil extract or essential oil, stop using it for at least two weeks before having surgery, because basil can increase bleeding. Speak to your doctor, nutritionist, or pharmacist before using basil if you are receiving treatment to lower your blood pressure.

Rhodiola

Rhodiola (*Rhodiola rosea*), also known as Aaron's rod and golden root, can be used to stimulate focus and memory. It is used as a traditional remedy to treat anxiety and fatigue in Scandinavia and Russia. The cognitive benefits of rhodiola were shown in a study that found a single dose improved memory and relieved depression (Palmeri et al., 2016).

When buying a rhodiola supplement, check the label or ask your pharmacist to make sure that it was tested by a third party. If a reputable third party such as NSF and USP has put its seal on the product label, this indicates that the supplement really contains what the label claims. Also, look for supplements that contain the same proportions of active ingredients that are found naturally in rhodiola roots, which are 3% rosavin and 0.8–1% salidroside.

Don't take your rhodolia supplement close to bedtime since it might keep you awake. The dosage will depend on the supplement manufacturer and generally ranges between 100 and 300 mg daily.

Rhodiola supplements might cause side effects such as difficulty falling asleep, dry mouth, and jitters. Because of the risk of negative interactions with certain conditions and medications, it is safer to avoid rhodiola if you have bipolar disorder, insomnia, or anxiety, or are taking stimulants.

Lifestyle Habits for a Happy Brain

The easiest way to keep your brain happy is to keep it active. Here are some activities to help your brain stay in shape:

- **Memory games.** These types of games stimulate areas in the brain responsible not only for recall but also for pattern recognition.
- **Do a jigsaw puzzle.** If you regularly do jigsaw puzzles, you are helping to protect your brain against aging effects as well as exercising your brain's memory, reasoning, and pattern recognition abilities.
- **Sodoku.** Playing sudoku is a fun way to challenge your brain. Sudoku puzzles range from easy to very difficult, so it is easy to find the level you enjoy most. To keep your brain sharp, try some more difficult levels than those you are used to.

- **Meditation.** The more you practice focused attention meditation, the more you train your brain to keep your concentration on a single task.
- **Chess.** You don't have to be a grand master to enjoy a friendly game. Chess can help keep your memory sharp and stimulate your ability to adapt your thinking to new situations.
- **Computer games.** Whether you play on your phone, TV, console, or computer, your brain enjoys the stimulation that games bring. Action games may quicken your reflexes, while strategy and puzzle games can help you develop your ability to strategize, keep your focus, and be flexible and adaptable with your problem-solving skills.
- **Learn something new.** Studying stimulates the formation of new neural connections and stimulates the blood supply to the brain.

Key Takeaways

When your estrogen levels start to decline, your brain has to get used to a different hormonal environment. This can lead to problems with memory and cognition, and, if you have these problems, you might worry about neurological disorders. Your doctor can help you determine if your memory problems are menopause related. If menopause is to blame for your foggy thinking, you can do several things to help your brain keep sharp, but know that your brain will recover in time.

Chapter 8

Natural Remedies Versus HRT— Navigating Your Choices for Hormonal Balance

We discussed HRT in detail in the first chapter and have mentioned several natural remedies for various symptoms during the course of this book. In this chapter, we'll look at natural remedies that focus on helping keep hormones in balance, and what factors to consider when deciding between conventional HRT and natural remedies. Keep in mind that your body produces more hormones than just estrogen and progesterone and that these other hormones should also be in balance for optimal health.

Hormones affect so many bodily processes that one imbalance can have a domino effect. You can help restore hormonal balance by trying one or more of the methods discussed in this chapter. Keep in mind, though, that natural remedies or HRT treatments that work for other women might not work for you, since everybody is unique.

If you have any questions about the suitability of any method, speak to your doctor or pharmacist.

Natural Remedies for Hormonal Balance: Lifestyle

Protein

During menopause, the loss of estrogen has a domino effect on several bodily processes such as metabolism and weight control. By regularly consuming protein, you help your body make peptide hormones, which help regulate processes affected by lower estrogen levels. Because protein stimulates hormones that make you feel full and inhibit the hormone that fuels your appetite, having a protein-rich meal can help you with weight management.

Include protein in your diet by eating eggs, lentils, meat, fish, or poultry, or by taking a protein supplement such as a protein bar or protein shake.

Stabilize Your Insulin

A study has shown that there is a relationship between estrogen and insulin resistance (De Paoli et al., 2021). Menopausal women are more likely to develop an insensitivity to insulin.

Insulin regulates blood sugar levels by stimulating the cells to absorb blood sugar (glucose) after a meal. When there isn't enough insulin, or if a person is insulin resistant, the cells don't absorb glucose. The unabsorbed glucose can't be burned for energy and will be stored as fat instead. The pancreas has to pump out more and more insulin to lower blood sugar, which can result in type 2 diabetes.

To keep your body sensitive to insulin, you can reduce your sugar intake. Many foods contain added sugars because they add texture and taste and prolong shelf life. Even savory foods such as instant beef soup or noodles can contain added sugar, especially in the form of high-fructose corn syrup. Read the labels of products to make sure you keep your sugar intake as low as possible.

You can also try these methods to maintain healthy insulin levels:

- Intermittent fasting will give your body the opportunity to lower insulin levels.
- Cut out processed foods since they are generally high in glucose.
- Keep your insulin receptors functioning by eating magnesium-rich foods or taking a magnesium supplement.
- Fiber affects how fast your body digests food. By eating sufficient fiber, digestion is slowed down and glucose is released less quickly. This prevents a sharp spike in blood sugar and a resulting spike in insulin.
- Exercise regularly to burn glucose energy.
- Eat foods rich in omega-3 fatty acids to help your cells become more sensitive to insulin.

Maintain a Healthy Weight

Because the loss of estrogen affects metabolism and fat distribution, the risk of obesity increases during menopause. Studies have shown that obesity is conducive to insulin resistance (Barazzoni et al., 2018). This can culminate in type 2 diabetes and more weight gain.

Fat cells produce can produce hormones, and one of these hormones, called leptin, helps to control appetite. Obese people can have high leptin levels, but their bodies tend to be insensitive to its effect, causing them to eat and not feel full.

Obesity can also lead to low levels of growth hormone. Because growth hormone plays a part in regulating metabolism, being obese can slow the metabolism down, which can lead to more weight gain.

Obesity can be reversed and, with it, insulin insensitivity. In Chapter 9, we'll discuss weight management in detail.

Take Care of Your Thyroid

Due to hormonal changes during menopause or other health factors, you might develop a condition where your thyroid gland isn't as active as it is supposed to be. This condition, where the thyroid is underactive, is called hypothyroidism. The thyroid gland plays an important part in regulating metabolism, and if it is underactive, metabolism slows down. People with hypothyroidism find it very difficult to lose weight.

It is also possible to have an imbalance in your thyroid hormones. When the thyroid hormones called T3 and T4 are out of balance, it can result in the body retaining salt and water, which leads to gaining water weight.

Thyroid hormones also play a part in regulating the hormones responsible for making you hungry and telling you when you are full. If levels of thyroid hormones are low, you may constantly feel hungry or not feel full after a big meal.

If you have a sluggish thyroid gland, there are things you can do to help you lose weight:

- **Increase your protein intake.** Lean protein can help stimulate your metabolism and make you feel full.
- **Hydrate.** Drinking enough water can help reduce water retention and appetite, and improve your digestion.
- **Don't cut too many calories.** It can be tempting to eat only low-calorie foods and live off a diet of black coffee and lettuce leaves, but although it might help you lose weight in the short term, you might end up with nutritional deficiencies that can cause serious health issues. Your thyroid gland needs nutrients

such as protein and iodine to produce thyroid hormones. Also, if your body doesn't get enough calories to fuel its necessary processes, it will go into starvation mode, which will burn muscle instead of fat.

- **Feel full with healthy fats.** Stay away from processed oils and eat salmon, tuna, mackerel, flaxseeds, and nuts instead. Not only will healthy fats keep you feeling comfortably full, but foods with healthy fats generally also contain selenium, which is needed for the thyroid gland to function at its best.

- **Go easy on the goitrogens.** Goitrogens are substances in some foods that can interfere with thyroid gland function. If you eat large amounts of goitrogens, your thyroid gland can struggle to regulate your metabolism, body temperature, blood calcium levels, and heart rate. Goitrogenic foods include corn, peanuts, linseed, strawberries, peaches, sweet potatoes, broccoli, cabbage, kale, pears, turnips, cauliflower, and soy-based foods.

- **Stop smoking.** Smoking increases the risk of the thyroid gland becoming less active.

- **Eat more iodine-rich foods.** Your thyroid can't function properly if it doesn't get sufficient amounts of iodine. Use iodized salt to season your food, or take a kelp supplement.

Exercise

Hormones work when they lock into special receptors. Exercise helps to make these receptors more sensitive to hormones such as insulin. Just like estrogen and progesterone, other hormones also drop off naturally as we age. These hormones include growth hormone (HGH), IGF-1, testosterone, and DHEA. A study has shown that exercise can help increase these hormones (Sato & Iemitsu, 2015). We'll discuss the value of movement during menopause in detail in Chapter 10.

Natural Remedies for Hormonal Balance: Herbal Supplements

Chaste Tree

Chaste tree (*Vitexagnus castus*), also known as *Vitex*, may stimulate the production of progesterone and lower levels of the hormone prolactin, which plays a part in PMS. A chaste berry supplement can help perimenopausal women who are estrogen dominant have a better hormonal balance, which can help alleviate PMS symptoms such as breast tenderness.

The potential side effects of chaste berry supplements are headache, diarrhea, menstrual changes, acne, dizziness, and fatigue. Because chaste tree affects hormones involved with menstruation, it isn't a suitable supplement for women who are trying to get pregnant, are pregnant, or are using oral birth control.

If you take medications to treat Parkinson's disease or take an antipsychotic drug, speak to your pharmacist before you try chaste berry because the supplement can make your medication less effective.

Alfalfa

Alfalfa (*Medicago sativa*) is used in traditional medicine to help treat not only hormonal irregularities but also arthritis, diabetes, and urinary tract infections. It helps relieve symptoms of menopause and PMS due to isoflavones, which are a type of phytoestrogen. It can also trigger the hormones that regulate the breast's milk glands and can stimulate the production of breast milk.

If you plan to use an alfalfa supplement, be aware that its high fiber content can cause diarrhea and flatulence. Supplements such as alfalfa that contain phytoestrogens aren't suitable for women who have or have had a hormone-sensitive condition such as uterine or breast cancer.

Alfalfa might exacerbate certain conditions. If you have rheumatoid arthritis, lupus, or multiple sclerosis, speak to your doctor or pharmacist before trying an alfalfa supplement. There is also a possibility that alfalfa can interact with medications used to treat high blood sugar, immunosuppressants, blood thinners, and medication that increases sensitivity to sunlight. Speak to your pharmacist about possible interactions if you are using prescription medication or are using other supplements and herbal remedies.

Burdock Root

A study on senior women with metabolic syndrome found that burdock increased their estrogen and DHEA hormone levels. Metabolic syndrome isn't unusual among menopausal women, and this condition is characterized by weight gain around the abdomen and high cholesterol, blood pressure, and blood sugar (Ha et al., 2018). The findings suggest that burdock root (*Arctium lappa*) can help reduce the menopause belly and contribute to better overall health.

Burdock root can have potential side effects such as high blood sugar, skin rash, and a possibility of causing jaundice. Fortunately, side effects of burdock root are generally rare.

There might be negative interactions if you use burdock root and diuretics, medications to treat diabetes, and tamoxifen, cisplatin, or quercetin cancer drugs. Burdock root might also interact with certain medications, so consult your doctor or pharmacist if you'd like to try burdock root while using these medications. If you are allergic to daisies or chrysanthemums, you are probably allergic to burdock as well.

Shatavari

Shatavari (*Asparagus racemosus*) isn't just used to help maintain collagen and keep the skin elastic. Practitioners of Ayurvedic medicine use shatavari as a tonic and a hormone balancer. A clinical review has concluded that shatavari can help treat hormone imbalance and, by extension, some conditions caused by hormonal imbalances, such as PCOS and infertility (Pandey et al., 2018).

Side effects from shatavari generally only occur due to an asparagus allergy and include symptoms such as difficulty breathing, rapid heart rate, skin rash, itchiness, and dizziness. There is also an increased risk of dehydration because shatavari acts as a diuretic.

Because shatavari can affect blood sugar and act as a diuretic, it should be avoided if you use any other diuretic or blood sugar herbal remedy or medication.

Dong Quai

This Asian herb is used in traditional Chinese medicine to treat menopause symptoms and restore hormonal balance. Dong quai (*Angelica sinensis*) contains phytoestrogens that have the same effect as estrogen, which can help balance the hormones of progesterone-dominant women. For more information, refer back to Chapter 1, where we discussed progesterone and estrogen dominance.

Dong quai can have some side effects, such as skin that is more sensitive to sunlight, increased blood pressure, and gas. Because dong quai can affect blood clotting, it isn't suitable for people who are taking blood thinners, have a bleeding disorder, or have surgery scheduled within the next two weeks.

There haven't been any studies to determine if it is safe to take dong quai for more than six months, so it is a good idea to speak to your pharmacist if you plan to take it long term.

Evening Primrose Oil

The high fatty acid content of evening primrose oil (*Oenothera biennis*) can help regulate the production of the hormone-like substances prostaglandins. Prostaglandins play a role in maintaining hormonal balance. Evening primrose oil can also help relieve hot flashes and increase progesterone production in estrogen-dominant women.

Side effects of evening primrose oil are rare but may include diarrhea, headache, nausea, skin rash, or dizziness. Side effects can be more intense for people who are using psychiatric medicines. Evening primrose oil can also increase the risk of bleeding for people who take anticoagulants.

HRT

HRT can help relieve several symptoms of menopause, especially in women whose symptoms are severe or who prefer the convenience of HRT over natural remedies. There are different types of HRT available, each with its own benefits and potential side effects.

We'll kick off this section by examining what HRT can do for you:

- **Improve bone density.** A study on pre- and postmenopausal women found that the transdermal estrogen patch improved their bone mineral density (Prestwood et al., 2003).
- **Treat depression due to hormonal fluctuations.** A study has shown that transdermal estrogen patches can relieve depression in perimenopausal women (Gordon & Girdler, 2014).

- **Help prevent age-related neurological conditions.** A meta-analysis has found that estrogen-based HRT can help protect against developing Alzheimer's disease and Parkinson's disease (Song et al., 2020).

Types of HRT

HRT is available in estrogen-only and estrogen and progestin combination forms, and it can take the form of skin patches (transdermal patches), tablets, topical gels and creams, and vaginal rings and suppositories. In this section, we'll take a closer look at the types of HRT.

Transdermal Patches

The patches that stick to the skin are categorized according to their ingredients:

- low-dose estrogen patches (these patches aren't used to treat menopause symptoms but are used to reduce the risk of developing osteoporosis)
- estrogen (estradiol) and progestin (norethindrone) combination patches
- estrogen (estradiol) patches

A review has concluded that using the transdermal patch has a lower risk of developing gallbladder disease than taking an oral HRT (Liu, 2013).

Vaginal Rings and Suppositories

Vaginal rings and suppositories enable low-dose estrogen, or an estrogen–progestin combo, to be placed directly into the vagina to treat symptoms such as vaginal itchiness, dryness, or painful intercourse. The rings are made from soft plastic, and they have benefits for perimenopausal women as well. Perimenopausal women can use vaginal rings as a contraceptive. As a contraceptive, vaginal rings have the advantage over oral contraceptives of staying effective even if you have vomiting or diarrhea. Vaginal rings have to be replaced every one to three months, depending on the product.

On the plus side, most vaginal rings and suppositories deliver only a low dose of estrogen, making it a safe option for women who can't take high-dose HRT. On the minus side, vaginal rings and suppositories that are low dose can only treat vaginal symptoms and no other menopausal malady. Women who haven't had a hysterectomy are advised to use vaginal rings and suppositories only short term to reduce the risk of uterine cancer.

Topical Estrogen Gel, Cream and Spray

Topical treatments are rubbed or sprayed onto the skin, from where they are absorbed into the bloodstream. Topical HRT is ideal for women who have high cholesterol or liver disease and is easy to apply. However, topical treatments can rub or wash off before they are completely absorbed and might have the same risks of negative effects as oral HRT.

Oral HRT

Of all the types of HRT, oral therapies have been studied the most, which means that your doctor can guide you through all the benefits and risks to help you decide if oral HRT is the treatment for you. Oral HRT can lead to side effects such as tender and swollen breasts, nausea, fluid retention, headache, and vaginal discharge. Oral HRT isn't suitable for women who have liver damage or high cholesterol.

Note that oral HRT isn't the same as oral birth control. Although they may contain the same synthetic hormones, the dosages are different. It is also possible for a perimenopausal woman to be on both HRT and birth control.

The Risks of HRT

Up until 2020, many menopausal women were wary of HRT, and for good reason. The Women's Health Initiative study, released in 2002, found that combining estrogen with progestin (synthetic progesterone) in HRT didn't improve cognition in postmenopausal women over 65 but instead increased the risk of developing dementia. The study also found that using estrogen derived from horse urine decreased the risk of hip fractures but increased the risk of having a stroke (Chlebowski & Aragaki, 2023). Menopausal women and their doctors started to doubt if HRT was worth it, especially since taking estrogen also increased the risk of recurrence of hormone-sensitive breast and uterine cancer.

The chemical composition of HRT is now more refined compared to the HRT that was available for the 2002 study. However, HRT can still increase the risk of developing gallbladder disease, breast and uterine cancer, blood clots, stroke, and heart attack. (Taking estrogen with progestin lowers the risk of uterine cancer, while estrogen-only increases the risk.) Women over 60 have the highest risk of getting these conditions due to HRT.

To minimize the risks of HRT, your doctor will start your treatment at the lowest dosage and re-evaluate every three to six months.

Other Pharmaceutical Treatments for Menopause Symptoms

If you want relief from certain menopause symptoms but don't want to use either HRT or herbal remedies, you can speak to your doctor about using some off-label medications. Here are a few that might help you during your menopause journey.

Clonidine

Clonidine is a type of medication used to treat high blood pressure. Your doctor might prescribe clonidine to ease hot flashes if nothing else has brought you relief. Clonidine might cause some side effects such as changes in heart rate and blood pressure, sleep issues, dizziness, and headache.

Antidepressants

Your doctor might prescribe a low-dose antidepressant called paroxetine to treat menopausal depression, mood swings, night sweats, and hot flashes. Paroxetine can cause some side effects such as headache, dry mouth, dizziness, and changes in sleeping patterns and sexual response.

Gabapentin

If your hot flashes are severe and you haven't found anything that effectively cools you down, your doctor might prescribe the anticonvulsant gabapentin. There are possible side effects when you use gabapentin, including fever, nausea, tremors, and vomiting.

Nonhormonal Vaginal Treatments

HRT isn't for everyone, and herbal remedies might take time to fully work. An alternative to HRT and herbs for vaginal issues during menopause is OTC vaginal moisturizers and lubricants. OTC means you can find these at your local pharmacy without a prescription. Your pharmacist can give you more details about products such as K-Y jelly, almond oil, and Replens.

Key Takeaways

When you seek help with your hormones during menopause, you don't have to take the first product suggested to you. You can choose whether you want a natural product, a prescription pharmaceutical, or an OTC remedy. There are also lifestyle adjustments you can make that will calm the hormonal storm and benefit your overall health as well.

Remember that you are unique, and you don't have to put up with a product that doesn't work for you. Your doctor and pharmacist are trained to help you find something that will make your menopause journey smooth sailing, so don't hesitate to speak to them if you have any questions.

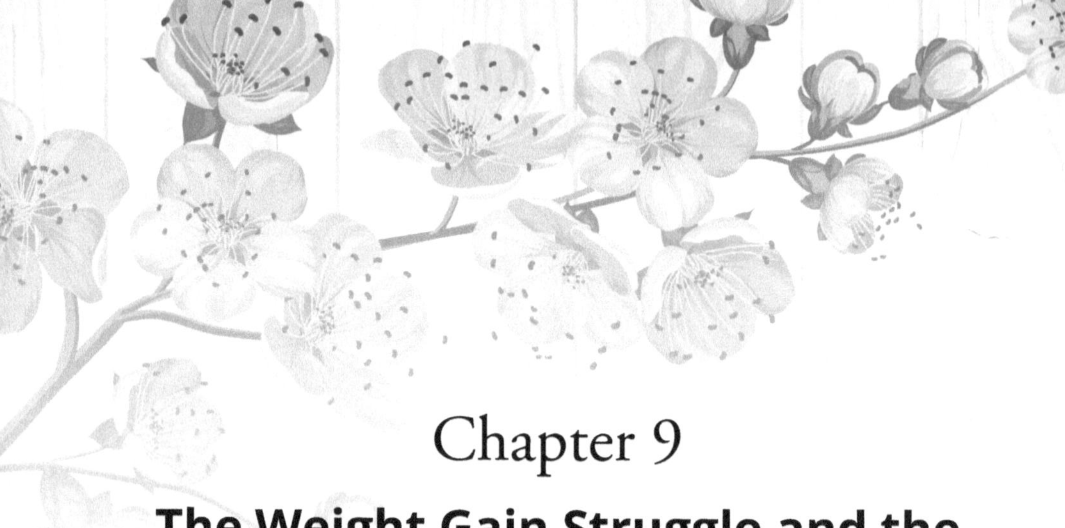

Chapter 9

The Weight Gain Struggle and the Metabolic Shift—Diet Adjustments for Hormonal Harmony

Meet Mary, a 61-year-old who has had enough of carrying extra weight on her bones. Mary used to think she started gaining weight in her late 40s because she was just unlucky to come from a family of large women. On her birthday, her best friend gave her a book about menopause. At first, Mary had no interest in reading it. Why would she, when her periods stopped almost 15 years ago?

However, Mary dug the book from the back of her closet after seeing a doctor on TV explain that many women tend to gain weight during menopause and that this weight gain puts them at risk of diabetes, heart disease, and osteoporosis. She discovered that menopausal weight gain is real and that it doesn't have to be permanent. Understanding menopausal weight gain enabled Mary to see what she needed to do to speed up her metabolism and shed the extra pounds. You can lose weight more easily too if you understand what's going on inside your body.

Even if you exercise regularly and avoid fast food as much as you can, you might find your waistline expanding from perimenopause onward. You might notice other weight issues that you never had to deal with before, such as gaining weight easily, difficulty losing weight, and having fat in body areas that used to be slim. In this chapter, we'll tackle menopausal weight gain and see what you can do to manage your weight.

What Is Menopausal Weight Gain?

Your body changes the calories from food into energy, which is a process called metabolism. Falling estrogen levels during menopause can lead to lower muscle mass. Muscle uses energy, and with lower lean muscle mass, less energy is used and more energy is left over, which your body can store as fat. This causes your metabolism to slow down. The slower your metabolism, the fewer calories you need to maintain your ideal weight.

Many women find that during menopause, they are more prone to gain weight around the midsection. Menopause is the time when women are likely to get a "jelly belly," which is notoriously difficult to get rid of. The reason it is more difficult to lose weight during menopause is that you need fewer calories to stay the same weight, and also that certain exercises can lead to weight gain!

The Consequences of Hormonal Weight Gain

Gaining weight around the abdomen can lead to a higher risk of certain health conditions. This is because abdominal fat isn't just under the skin, but also around the internal organs. The fat you can pinch under the skin is called subcutaneous fat, and the fat surrounding the organs is called visceral fat. Because fat distribution changes during menopause, even women who don't gain a lot of weight can have visceral fat.

Metabolic syndrome is a set of health conditions such as high blood pressure, insulin resistance, and high cholesterol. Metabolic syndrome increases your risk of suffering heart disease, diabetes, or stroke. Visceral fat is a symptom of metabolic syndrome. So, if your visceral fat increases, so does your chance of developing metabolic syndrome.

Visceral fat not only increases your odds of stroke, gallbladder disease, heart disease, and type 2 diabetes, but also of the following medical conditions:

- osteoarthritis
- liver disease
- gout
- cancer
- lumbago (pain in the lower back)
- asthma
- dementia

Visceral fat causes a higher risk of the above conditions because this type of fat produces special proteins that increase inflammation and can narrow blood vessels.

A rough guideline to see if you have visceral fat is to measure your waistline. Take your waist circumference around the widest part of your belly without sucking in your stomach or tightening the measuring tape. If you are Asian, you probably have a visceral fat issue if your waist measurement is 31.5 inches or more (35.5 inches for Asian men). If you aren't of Asian descent, a waist circumference of 35 inches or more indicates visceral fat (40 inches for men).

If you want to know exactly how much visceral fat you have, your doctor can order an imaging test. These tests can be expensive, and it is much cheaper to focus on weight management, which can benefit you in the long run.

Managing Weight

To lose weight, you require a calorie deficit; in other words, you have to burn more calories than you ingest. You can achieve this in two ways: ingest fewer calories per day or exercise more. Ideally, you should aim for a combination of more movement and fewer calories. The combination will help you lose weight faster than either method alone.

An easy first step to reduce calorie intake is to keep an eye out for added sugars. Many products, from bread to gravy, contain added sugar, which is very calorie dense. Even foods that don't taste sweet might have sugar as an ingredient. Sugar adds taste, helps baked goods to brown, and acts as a preservative. Often, manufacturers hide sugar content by renaming sugar.

If a label lists any of the following, there is added sugar under a hidden name:

- sucrose
- cane juice crystals
- cane syrup
- evaporated cane syrup
- high-fructose corn syrup
- ethyl maltol
- sorghum
- galactose
- glucose
- dextrose
- dextran
- malt
- maltodextrin
- molasses
- blackstrap molasses
- brown rice sugar

- agave nectar
- maple syrup
- golden syrup
- coconut sugar
- raw sugar
- fructose

Where Does the Fat Go?

When you diet or exercise, you might notice parts of your body getting smaller. You realize that your body's fat stores are shrinking. Have you ever wondered where the fat goes and how it leaves your body?

Fat cells are called adipocytes. Everyone has billions of adipocytes, and these fat cells can vary in size. Because fat is necessary for certain bodily functions, even the most lean athlete doesn't have 0% body fat. There are two types of fat in your body: white and brown adipocytes. The brown fat cells help to regulate your body temperature by burning calories. Brown adipocytes contain many droplets of fat plus water, salts, mitochondria, and protein. Mitochondria are little organelles that transform calories from food into energy. White fat cells contain only a single droplet of fat and some protein, water, and salts.

When fat is burned to provide energy or heat, the fat cells shrink. The chemical process that causes fat to release energy also causes fatty acids to be converted into water and carbon dioxide. The carbon dioxide is exhaled and the water is excreted in urine.

To lose a pound of fat, you need to burn 3,500 calories. This is more than an average woman or man needs daily to maintain weight. Cutting calories off your daily intake will add up, and you can easily lose a pound a week with a healthy lifestyle. You can also exercise the pounds away. It takes about 10 hours of squats or six hours of high-intensity interval training (HIIT) to lose a pound of fat. Of course, any exercise will burn calories, but you have to do it consistently.

The Stages of Weight Loss

Many people who've been on diets lose weight fast in the beginning and then may reach a plateau of no weight loss, followed by slow weight loss. These variations in weight loss speed are normal, and happen because the body loses weight in stages.

During the first stage of weight loss, you tend to lose weight fairly fast. During the first month or two of a weight-loss program, your body loses mass mostly from stored carbohydrates, water, and protein. Fat is burned as well, but doesn't account for the majority of the weight loss. If your weight-loss diet cuts carbs, your carb stores will run empty faster and you'll lose weight faster.

In the second stage, your body will burn mostly fat. You will lose weight more slowly and can experience plateaus as a result of your body adjusting its metabolism to burn fewer calories; it does this because your body doesn't like losing its fat reserves. Our bodies are adapted for survival, and fat reserves can help us survive a famine, which is why your metabolism slows down at some points during a diet. If you put your body in starvation mode by following a too-low-calorie diet, the weight loss can slow down to a snail's pace as your body tries to protect itself.

Natural Remedies to Facilitate Weight Loss

If you take a natural remedy to help you lose weight, you have control over the dosage and you know exactly what you are putting into your body. There are some natural remedies that you may already have in your kitchen. In this section, we'll take a look at some commonly available remedies to kick-start your weight loss.

Cinnamon

Because cinnamon may boost metabolism, it can help you burn more calories. To get a daily dose of fat-burning cinnamon, mix a teaspoon of cinnamon with the juice of half a lemon (or a teaspoon of concentrated lemon juice) into a glass of hot water, and drink it on an empty stomach.

Green Tea

Two ingredients of green tea, caffeine and catechins, can help you lose weight. Drinking a cup of green tea two to three times per day can accelerate your weight loss.

Oolong Tea

Oolong tea can help accelerate your metabolism and reduce the formation of fat cells. It can also help you keep off the pounds if you are prone to gaining weight after a diet. Make oolong tea by steeping a teaspoon of oolong tea in a cup of hot water for 10 minutes before straining the tea.

Ginger

Ginger tea can help you feel more full between meals. Add ginger to your weight management arsenal by steeping a teaspoon of grated ginger in a cup of hot water for 10 minutes.

Cayenne Pepper

The capsaicin that gives cayenne pepper its bite can raise body temperature and switch metabolism into a higher gear. If you prefer not to sprinkle cayenne pepper over your food, you can mix a teaspoon (or half a teaspoon if you aren't used to the taste) of cayenne pepper into a glass of water and drink the mixture once daily.

Yogurt

Metabolism and digestion can become sluggish after menopause. One way to stimulate digestion is to eat probiotics to provide food for your helpful intestinal bacteria. Yogurt is a good probiotic, and your improved digestion can also give your metabolism a boost.

Prescription Diet Pills

If you meet certain medical criteria, you could benefit from certain FDA-approved drugs to help you lose weight. Weight loss drugs, also known as slimming or diet pills, are designed to help with weight loss, but you'll still need to watch your diet and exercise regularly to get the best, healthiest results. In this section, we'll take an informative look at pharmaceutical weight loss aids.

Saxenda

Saxenda (liraglutide) is an injection that suppresses appetite and increases feelings of fullness. It is used to help people who have a BMI higher than 30, or a BMI between 27 and 30 who also have a medical condition made worse by their weight. Such conditions include high blood pressure and type 2 diabetes.

If you are interested in taking Saxenda, be aware of possible side effects, including headache, nausea, constipation, low blood sugar, and diarrhea. There is also a risk that Saxenda use might lead to acute pancreatitis, gallbladder disease, and very low blood sugar. Saxenda can't be used by women who are breastfeeding, are taking insulin, or have personal or a family history of thyroid cancer, or a disorder called multiple endocrine neoplasia syndrome type 2.

Xenical

Xenical (orlistat) reduces your body's ability to absorb fat. Instead of absorbing fat from food, the fat passes into the stool. Doctors can prescribe Xenical to people who are overweight and have conditions that could be better controlled if they lost weight, such as heart disease, high cholesterol, and diabetes.

To help reduce or prevent gastrointestinal side effects, it is best to follow a low-fat diet while taking Xenical. However, Xenical might still cause side effects such as stomach ache, loose stools, anxiety, headache, and, in perimenopausal women, irregular periods. Because Xenical blocks fat, it also blocks the absorption of fat-soluble vitamins, which can lead to vitamin deficiencies.

Phentermine

Phentermine (Lomaira, Suprenza, Adipex-P) is an appetite suppressant aimed at people with a minimum BMI of 30, or a BMI of 27 and higher if there is also a weight-related health problem.

Some side effects might occur, such as constipation, insomnia, dry mouth, nausea, and diarrhea. Phentermine isn't suitable for pregnant or breastfeeding women or people with glaucoma, overactive thyroid glands, or heart disease.

Wegovy

Wegovy (semaglutide) is an appetite suppressor given as an injection once a week. It is designed for people with a minimum BMI of 30, or a BMI of 27 with a medical condition such as high blood pressure, too much fat in the bloodstream (dyslipidemia), and diabetes.

Although Wegovy is an effective appetite suppressant, it isn't for everyone. It can cause several side effects, ranging from uncomfortable to serious, such as abdominal bloating, flatulence, constipation, vomiting, nausea, diarrhea, dizziness, indigestion, burping, headache, heart palpitations, gastroenteritis, severe allergic reaction, suicidal ideation, or a red, enlarged, bulbous nose in people with diabetes. Wegovy should also be avoided by people who are sensitive to semaglutide (an ingredient in Wegovy) or who have (or have a family history of) thyroid cancer or gland tumors. Wegovy isn't safe for perimenopausal women who are trying to become pregnant or are pregnant.

Qsymia

Qsymia contains phentermine, which we discussed previously, and topiramate. Both these ingredients are appetite suppressants, but phentermine works immediately while topiramate takes a while to be released, which leads to longer periods of not feeling hungry. Doctors can prescribe Qsymia to people with a BMI of 30 and more, or a BMI of 27 and above if there is also a weight-related health issue.

Qsymia isn't free of side effects and can cause insomnia, dry mouth, irritability, depression, blurry vision, constipation, tingly sensations in the skin, anxiety, depression, fatigue, and headaches. It can also make food taste different. Avoid Qsymia if you are pregnant because it increases the baby's risk of cleft palate or cleft lip.

Contrave

Contrave (naltrexone HCl/bupropion HCl) works in two ways: It suppresses appetite, and causes more calories to be burned. It is suitable for people with a BMI of 30 and up, or a BMI of 27 and above if there is also a medical condition that will be relieved with weight loss.

Side effects of Contrave include vomiting, dry mouth, nausea, insomnia, headache, constipation, and diarrhea. This diet pill can also cause an increased risk of liver damage, mania, seizures, rapid heart rate, increased blood pressure, vision problems, and low blood sugar. When first starting to take Contrave, there is a risk of suicidal ideation.

Over-the-Counter Weight-Loss Supplements

Weight-loss supplements aren't regulated by the FDA. When you buy a weight-loss supplement, look at the label or ask your pharmacist if the product was tested by a reputable third party. Third-party testing can make sure that the ingredients listed on the label are really in the product, in the quantities stated. Let's explore some of the more popular OTC weight-loss supplements on the market.

Glucomannan

Glucomannan is generally not sold by itself but as an ingredient in a supplement. Glucomannan, which is a dietary fiber, changes into a gel-like substance in the stomach. This gel prevents the stomach from emptying quickly, thus making you feel fuller for longer. To prevent toxic or allergic reactions to glucomannan, consume less than 3 g daily.

There might be some side effects if you take glucomannan, such as bloating, diarrhea, belching, and constipation.

Some supplements combine glucomannan with *Garcinia cambogia* to facilitate even more weight loss.

Raspberry Ketones

Manufacturers of raspberry ketones claim that they can help break down fat, speed up metabolism, and reduce the amount of fat stored. Taking raspberry ketones can lead to side effects such as jitteriness, a faster heart rate, and higher blood pressure. There is also a possibility that raspberry ketones can cause a sudden constriction of the heart arteries called a coronary vasospasm. Avoid raspberry ketones if you are pregnant, breastfeeding, or taking blood thinners.

Chromium Picolinate

Chromium picolinate (or chromium) may act as an appetite suppressant and stimulate the body to burn more calories. Side effects are rare since chromium is an essential nutrient, but can include vertigo, watery stools, headache, nausea, hives, and constipation.

Chromium supplements aren't suitable for people who are also taking medications for thyroid conditions or diabetes.

Meratrim

Meratrim contains extracts that might have an appetite-suppressing effect and may play a role in lowering levels of unhealthy cholesterol. Meratrim can cause mania, liver damage, or serotonin toxicity, but these effects are extremely rare.

Alli

Alli is the toned-down, OTC version of the prescription weight loss drug Xenical, which we discussed earlier. The difference between Xenical and Alli is that Alli contains a lower dosage of the active ingredient. Just like Xenical, Alli interferes with fat absorption and has the same side effects. However, you don't need a prescription for Alli, and it is suitable for people with a BMI of 25 or more.

If you've had an organ transplant, are pregnant or breastfeeding, have a condition that affects the way your food absorbs nutrients, or are taking anticoagulants, cyclosporine, or antiretrovirals, Alli isn't a safe supplement for you.

Green Coffee Bean Extract

Green coffee, also known as raw coffee, can suppress appetite and reduce fat storage. The only reported side effects are headache and urinary tract infections, and green coffee bean extract is considered safe for everyone. If you have any concerns about the safety of this weight loss aid, speak to your doctor or pharmacist.

Hoodia

Hoodia is an herbal extract appetite suppressant that might help people with a metabolic disease lose weight. Metabolic diseases are caused by abnormal metabolic processes and include conditions such as type 2 diabetes, maple syrup urine disease, Tay-Sachs disease, and a build-up of too much iron (hemochromatosis).

Hoodia might cause certain side effects such as strange sensations in the skin, nausea, vomiting, and dizziness. People who have blood pressure problems, bile duct or gallbladder conditions, or impaired heart function might experience a worsening of symptoms. Speak to your doctor or pharmacist if you want to take hoodia but have any of the aforementioned health conditions.

Forskolin

Forskolin is a plant extract that is marketed as a carb blocker. It is especially suitable for people with insulin resistance. There are some potential side effects, including loose stools and more frequent bowel movements. Forskolin isn't suitable for people with polycystic kidney disease.

Before You Buy

If you plan to use an OTC or herbal weight-loss supplement, you must consider if the product will be suitable for you. In the previous sections, we noted that some supplements can be a health risk if you have certain medical conditions or use specific medications.

When you are in the process of picking a supplement, read the label or package insert, or consult your pharmacist to find out if it is safe to take a product if you

- use prescription medications, supplements (even vitamin pills), or herbal remedies
- have a personal or family history of a medical condition
- are breastfeeding, pregnant, or want to become pregnant
- are allergic, or potentially allergic, to any ingredient in the product

Why Fad and Starvation Diets Don't Work Long Term

In order to lose weight, you need to burn more calories than you consume. If weight loss is so easy, then every diet that restricts calories should be fine—but unfortunately, some diets can have detrimental effects on your health.

Every couple of years, a new fad diet hits the kitchens of millions of hopefuls across the world—diets that consist only of protein, no protein, high carbs, and no carbs, all of them promising that the diet is science based, healthy, and will melt pounds away faster than a donut disappears the day before starting a diet. These diets are known as fad diets. Some of them do result in weight loss, but they are anything but healthy. We'll take a look at some fad diets and the reasons they aren't long-term solutions.

Detox Diets

You have probably seen or heard ads where a celebrity praised a detox diet and proclaimed that they lost a massive amount of weight in a short time after removing toxins from their bodies. The next time you hear such a claim, you can rest assured that you have an efficient, natural detox system already in place: your kidneys and liver. It is the job of these organs to remove toxins from your body, and they don't need a special diet to do their jobs. However, some detox diets can cleanse your intestinal system to a degree, but this is only temporary and often not as effective as advertised.

Gluten-Free Diets

There are health conditions that necessitate a gluten-free diet, such as wheat allergy, celiac disease, and non-celiac gluten sensitivity. Most healthy people don't need to follow a gluten-free diet and can even harm their health with such a diet. Gluten-free foods generally have more sugar and fat and therefore also contain more calories than the same food with gluten. Due to the higher calories, gluten-free diets can lead to insulin resistance and weight gain.

Keto Diet

The keto diet can effectively help you lose weight, and it is especially good for people with epilepsy who don't have positive results from standard epilepsy medications (*Ketogenic Diet (Keto Diet) for Epilepsy*, 2020). You don't have to do keto for long before you run the risk of getting the so-called "keto flu." The keto flu is a set of side effects of the diet and include constipation, nausea, headache, dizziness, constant fatigue, and a low exercise tolerance. Fortunately, these symptoms are temporary and go away on their own as your body adjusts to the diet. Staying on the keto diet long term can lead to more serious conditions than keto flu, such as kidney stones, various vitamin deficiencies, and fatty liver disease. Also, keto can be very harmful for people with type 1 diabetes.

Menopause Diet

Diet pills and herbal remedies are only supplements, which means that although they can accelerate weight loss, you still have to exercise and follow a diet that will give you a calorie deficit. For an ideal diet to lose menopause-related weight, help relieve symptoms, and maintain your overall health, follow these guidelines:

- Eat plant-based foods that are high in phytoestrogens, such as soy, broccoli, and berries.
- Take care of your bones with foods containing an abundance of vitamin D, calcium, and magnesium, such as dairy products, eggs, and leafy green vegetables.
- Include more fatty fish, flaxseeds, and chia seeds into your diet to help reduce hot flashes and take care of your heart health.
- Stay away from prepackaged, processed foods and refined carbs such as white rice, cookies, and pasta.

Exercises That Increase Fat

Yes, you read it right the first time. It is possible to sabotage your weight-loss efforts with exercise!

One type of exercise that can really help burn fat and increase fitness is called high-intensity interval training, or HIIT. The problem with HIIT, especially for perimenopausal and menopausal women whose hormonal state is changing, is that HIIT is stressful to the body. This stress can increase the levels of the hormone cortisol, and cortisol levels can remain high after exercise. That can be a good thing, since your body then ups its metabolism to provide energy for survival, which means that glucose levels rise and fat and carbs get broken down faster. However, too much cortisol, or a cortisol imbalance, can lead to chronically high cortisol, which can fire up the appetite, cause the body to burn muscle protein instead of fat for energy, contribute to water retention, and make you feel tired. A scientific study has shown that chronically high cortisol can be a cause of weight gain and belly fat, especially in lean women (Epel et al., 2000).

To avoid gaining weight due to exercise-induced high cortisol, you can rest for longer between workout sessions, have fewer workouts, and reduce your cortisol with relaxing activities such as meditation, tai chi, listening to soothing music, or doing yoga.

Lifestyle Adjustments

- **Get more sleep.** Not getting enough sleep can increase your ghrelin levels. Ghrelin is the hormone that makes you feel hungry. Sleep deprivation also reduces levels of the hormone called leptin, which suppresses appetite. Therefore, if you don't sleep well, you'll tend to feel hungry more often. It can be hard to get quality sleep when you are struggling with night sweats and insomnia. Speak to your doctor or pharmacist about sleep aids that won't leave you groggy the next day or lead to dependency.
- **Drink enough water.** Water can help you feel full and aids digestion. As an added bonus, your skin can look more hydrated and clear.

- **Be mindful.** If you tend to eat out of boredom or habit, or if you eat when you are feeling emotional, you might eat more than you need to maintain or lose weight. Focusing on the texture and appearance of food, and paying attention to the physical act of chewing while savoring the taste, can help you break the habit of eating when you aren't hungry.
- **Move more.** Your muscles need energy to move, and this energy comes from burned calories. Regular exercise is a good diet's best partner.

Key Takeaways

Understanding your body and the changes to your bodily processes during menopause can help you make changes to your lifestyle that can smooth your journey. The key is to do so in a healthy way, especially when you are trying to lose weight. Going on a fad diet or starving yourself isn't a good long-term strategy. Aim to optimize your health so that you can have a long, happy, fulfilling future to look forward to.

In the next chapter, we'll take a look at how exercise and mindfulness can boost your energy levels.

Chapter 10

Movement and Mindfulness— Exercise Essentials for Energy Boosting and Tranquility

The hormonal and metabolic changes that occur during menopause can take a toll on energy levels. Sometimes, especially after a busy day at work or a morning lounging around watching TV, exercise is the last thing on our minds. We know that we need to exercise to keep our hearts healthy, keep excess weight off, and protect our bones, but sometimes the motivation is lacking. So, what is the cure for fatigue and lack of motivation? Exercise! If you wonder how the thing you are trying to avoid can be helpful, read on.

Exercise, Energy, and Menopause

Although intense, demanding exercises such as HIIT can help you lose weight, if you overdo it or don't take enough time to rest between sessions, you might gain weight instead. This is because intense exercise puts the body under stress, causing a release of cortisol. Cortisol levels that stay high for long periods can cause fat storage instead of burning it.

Exercise will also give your metabolism a wake-up call. Menopause might have caused your metabolism to slow to a crawl, leading to difficulty losing weight and a general lack of energy. When you exercise more, your body will undergo changes to make more energy available.

The Connection Between Energy and Exercise

When you exercise, things happen on the cellular level. The more you exercise, the more your cells are stimulated to produce more mitochondria in muscles. Mitochondria are organelles in your cells that use glucose and oxygen to provide energy. Thus, exercising regularly causes your body to have more energy providers. Your body will also have more oxygen when you exercise. The more oxygen, the more the mitochondria can produce energy.

Where Does Your Energy Come From?

During digestion, your body uses enzymes to break food down and absorb the nutrients from the food. The nutrients get transported into the cells, where mitochondria combine glucose from food with oxygen to produce energy in the form of a chemical called adenosine triphosphate (ATP). It is ATP that is the fuel of your body's cells.

Exercise and Metabolism

Your body uses energy for the processes that keep you alive. The energy needed to fuel these bodily processes, such as your breathing and heartbeat, is called basal metabolism. Your basal metabolic rate is a measure of how fast your body uses energy for vital functions. Your basal metabolic rate depends on factors such as your weight, genetics, age, and sex. As we get on in years, our muscle mass naturally drops, and this also leads to a slowing down of basal metabolic rate.

Yoga and tai chi can help you restore your emotional balance and give you a sense of tranquility. This is due to the nature of these exercises; they focus on controlled, smooth movements, awareness of breathing and movement, and a still mind. The gentle exercises will also stimulate blood flow and give your metabolism a boost without placing excessive stress on the body.

If you want to try yoga or tai chi, you can join a class or a virtual class, or find tutorials online. Start slowly and, especially with yoga, don't force your muscles into positions or stretches they aren't used to. Do only what is comfortable, and as your body becomes more flexible, you'll be naturally able to hold a position or stretch for longer.

The exercises (except for the more advanced yoga poses) look deceptively easy, but they are challenging enough to benefit the body as well as the mind. You'll find yourself more flexible and toned, with better posture and less tense muscles.

Aerobic and Anaerobic Exercise

Aerobic exercise, also called cardio, is the type of exercise where you breathe faster and your heart rate goes up for a certain time. When you do aerobic exercise such as cycling or swimming, your body mainly uses oxygen as fuel.

Anaerobic exercises are maximum-effort movements that require quick energy bursts, such as lifting weights or sprinting. During anaerobic exercise, your body uses mainly stored energy for fuel instead of oxygen.

Both aerobic and anaerobic exercises are needed for a fully rounded exercise program, since each type has its own particular benefits.

What Aerobic Exercise Can Do for You

Aerobic exercises, such as rowing, brisk walking, jogging, cross-country skiing, dancing, and stair climbing, may offer you these benefits:

- increase stamina
- improve heart health
- improve immunity to illness
- lower blood pressure
- weight loss
- improve mood

What Anaerobic Exercise Can Do for You

Anaerobic exercises, including HIIT, calisthenics, power-lifting, and sprinting, may also do wonderful things to your body:

- increase bone strength
- build and strengthen muscle
- burn fat
- improve stamina

Supplements for Energy

Exercise, sufficient rest and sleep, and a healthy diet are essential for optimal energy levels. There may be times when you aren't able to get the nutrients, sleep, or exercise you need, and you may need a supplement to boost your energy. Here are a few supplements that can help lift your energy levels by boosting metabolism and supporting mitochondria:

- coenzyme Q-10
- vitamin K
- vitamin E
- acetyl coenzyme A (acetyl-A)
- vitamin B complex
- vitamin C
- carnitine (L-carnitine)
- arginine
- iodine
- magnesium
- iron

Some of these supplements are discussed in more detail in Chapters 7 and 9.

Getting Started

The key to an exercise routine that will give you all the benefits without injuries, sprains, and strains is to start slowly. Do enough that it makes a difference, but not so much that you risk tearing a muscle. Just like diet, moderation is important for exercise too.

When you start an exercise program, do the minimum recommended amount and gradually work your way up. As long as you challenge your body, your cells will use energy more efficiently, and your overall energy levels will rise as a result.

Draw up a weekly or monthly schedule and stick to it. If you find it difficult, partner with a friend or family member so that you don't exercise alone. This way, both of you are accountable and can support and encourage each other.

If you don't want to leave the house to exercise, or you don't have an exercise partner to keep you on track, consider joining an online exercise class. Some online fitness groups or classes offer meal plans, personalized exercise programs, and reminders.

Anxiety and Depression During Menopause

The brain is very sensitive to hormones. When hormones become imbalanced or drop to lower levels during menopause, it can trigger imbalances in other hormones and neurotransmitters. Serotonin and endorphins, responsible for making us feel good, drop. Epinephrine and cortisol, which make us feel anxious and cranky, rise. Without steady levels of progesterone and estrogen to mitigate the effects of these stress hormones, women can experience anxiety and depression.

If you have anxiety or depression, the first step is to speak to your doctor. Once you've gotten help from a medical professional, you can incorporate mindfulness meditation to help ease your mental state.

Before Melissa entered perimenopause, she was under the impression that anxiety was merely the butterflies in her tummy before an exam, job interview, or first date. In her mid-40s, Melissa started to experience anxiety that ranged from intense nervousness to feelings of sheer panic. The anxiety never seemed to stop. She woke up nervous and tense, and went to bed with feelings of dread that kept her awake. Melissa started to struggle at work. Concentrating became difficult, and her heart started pounding before meetings. She developed mild depression and was always on the verge of tears. Her teenage daughter convinced Melissa to see a doctor after she complained of chest pains and almost passed out during a panic attack.

Her doctor tested her hormone levels and announced that she was perimenopausal. The doctor explained that anxiety and depression can be a side effect of hormone fluctuations, prescribed her an antidepressant and HRT, and advised her to sign up for a yoga or mindfulness class. The class helped Melissa take back control of her mind, and the anxiety subsided. The antidepressants helped to restore her positive outlook on life.

In the next section, we'll discuss mindfulness meditation as a method to help overcome anxiety and depression. It is important to know that the following methods are not meant to replace medical help but to support it.

What Is Mindfulness Meditation?

Mindfulness is a mental practice where your focus is on the moment. You concentrate on your immediate environment and pay attention to your senses without hurry or judgment. This trains your mind to relax, to not be anxious about possible scenarios, and to become more focused and able to pay attention to the world around you. Mindfulness relaxes your body and mind, and this helps combat conditions such as insomnia, anxiety, stress, high blood pressure, and panic disorders.

Mindfulness Techniques

Below, we'll briefly explore some mindfulness techniques that you can do anytime you want.

Mindful Walking

It doesn't matter how far you walk as long as you walk slowly and focus on the act of walking. Become mindful of the sensations when your feet make contact with the ground and the feeling of your muscles during the movement. Listen to your breathing, and become aware of the subtle shifts in your ankles and arms needed to maintain your balance.

Body Scan

Although you can do a body scan in any position, lying down is easiest, especially if you are a newbie to mindfulness. All you have to do is lie down comfortably, on your back if you can, and start focusing on your toes. Pay attention to the feelings in your toes, then your feet, then your ankles. Move your mindful attention up slowly from your toes to the top of your head. If any thoughts intrude while you are scanning, note the thought but don't pay attention to it. Let the thought drift away and return your attention to your body scan. If you suddenly feel an itch or a twinge, you can have a quick scratch or rub, then put it out of your mind and continue scanning.

Breathing

All you have to do is breathe slowly and deeply, in a restful and controlled manner. Pay attention to the rise and fall of your lungs, and feel the air entering and leaving your body. Notice how your nose and throat feel when the air moves across them.

Key Takeaways

Exercise improves your body's manufacture and use of energy at the cellular level. The more you exercise, the more energy and stamina you'll have, and you'll enjoy other health benefits as well.

There are two main types of exercise, classified as aerobic and anaerobic, according to the primary source of energy used during the movements. If your body uses oxygen as fuel during sustained movements, it is called aerobic exercise. Exercise that requires intense bursts of energy uses glucose as fuel, which is called anaerobic. Include exercises from both types to get the best of both worlds.

For some women, the change in hormonal levels during menopause brings with it anxiety and depression. If you are one of these women, and anxiety, panic attacks, and depression are affecting your quality of life, speak to your doctor. There is treatment available. However, you can also practice mindfulness meditation as a supplement to your medication.

We've come near to the end of your journey through the trials and tribulations of menopause and what you can do to triumph over them. In the conclusion, we'll look at the silver linings of menopause.

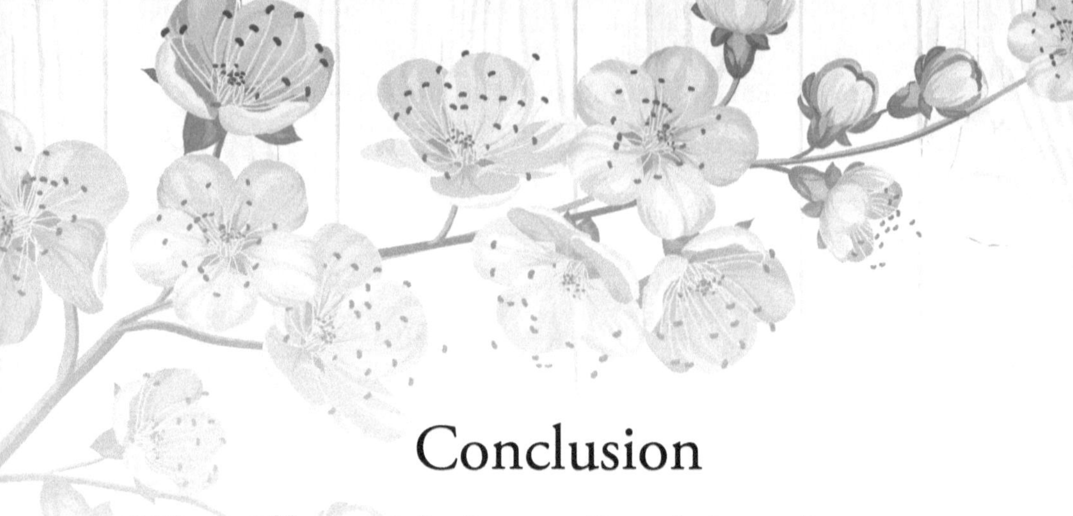

Conclusion

The Silver Lining—Positive Aspects of Post-Menopausal Life

When talking about menopause, the focus is often on the negative effects. We read and hear about the discomfort of night sweats, the frustration of hot flashes, the loss of libido, and the moodiness. But it is very seldom that we hear anyone mention the positives of menopause. So, let's break the mold and talk about the silver lining of being postmenopausal.

The shiniest silver lining is probably the freedom from menstruation. No more planning around your cycle; you can go anywhere you please at any time you want without worrying if you have to take tampons with you, or if you might leak. If you have cramps, imagine never having to grit your teeth through the pain every month.

Another silver lining of sweet freedom is being liberated from fertility. Motherhood can be a fantastic, fulfilling experience, but after a certain age, the idea of running after a toddler or dealing with a sulky teenager loses its appeal. Menopause frees you up from worrying about an unwanted pregnancy, and this can add spice and extra confidence to your bedroom adventures.

Menopause is a time of transition, and, like most changes, it can be challenging and uncomfortable. It is a time when you are growing into yourself, into the total of your experiences, wisdom, and potential. Your body starts redirecting energy from your body into your spirit and rewards you with the ability to see things without the cloudy vision of societal expectations.

Dealing with menopause symptoms focuses your attention on self-care. It is time to prioritize your own health and well-being. Your lifestyle might need adjustment, and your mind might need to let go of stresses and concerns that aren't needed anymore. Your food shouldn't be for the sake of convenience anymore, but for nourishment, and your exercises not for the sake of appearance, but for health and longevity.

Remember that there is no other woman like you; no one has ever had your unique experiences and thoughts, and no one has your unique genetic combination and biochemistry. Therefore, you have to forge your own unique path and use the remedies that work for you. If something works for your sister but not for you, discard it and try something different.

You can pioneer your own path, but you don't have to do it alone. There might be times when you mourn the loss of your fertility or gray-free hair, or feel anxious about the future. It is normal and natural. When your day is rough and your mood is low, lean on others. Speak to a loved one, a mental health professional, or a support group. You might be surprised how liberating it can be to give voice to your troubles, and how much lighter you feel afterwards. Also, keep in mind that your doctor and pharmacist are trained to give you advice, and are knowledgeable about everything menopause related. They've heard many other women speak about the same symptoms you might be having, so you can be open and honest about your symptoms and concerns. They are professionals who won't laugh or judge, but who will help in whatever capacity they can.

As a final word of encouragement, know that aging is a process that can add grace, empowerment, and serenity. Don't be afraid of menopause, but embrace it as the portal to a new and exciting chapter of your life. Know that the symptoms will pass and that there are many new beginnings, new challenges, and good things waiting for you.

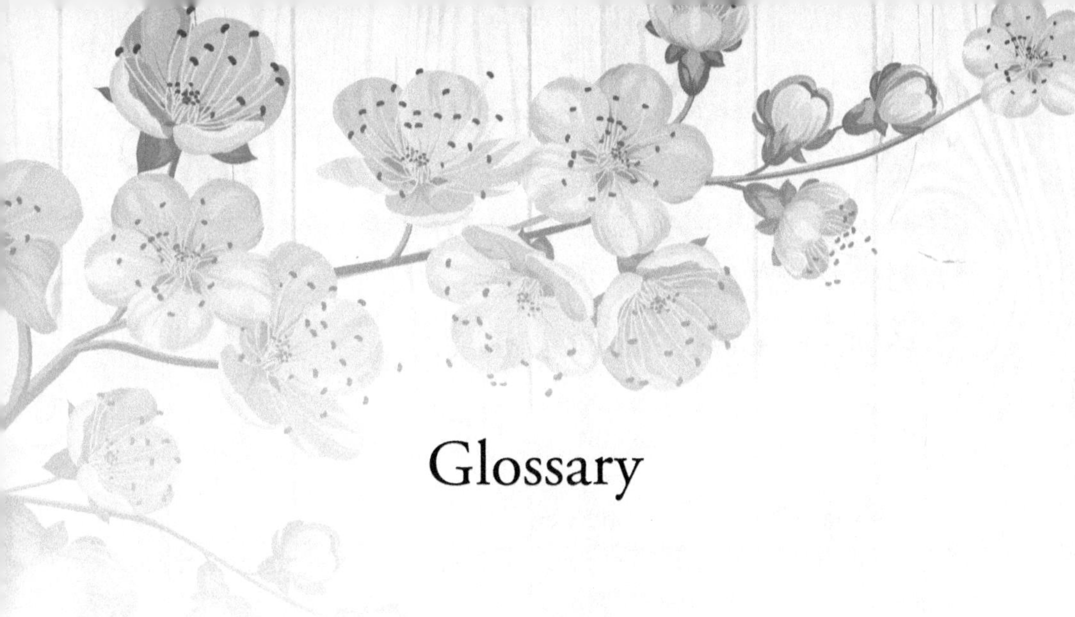

Glossary

Brain fog: Difficulty concentrating and thinking clearly.

Estrogen: The primary female hormone.

Hormone replacement therapy (HRT): Medical treatment involving synthetic estrogen and progesterone to increase levels of these hormones.

Hypothalamus: The part of the brain that produces certain hormones that regulate body temperature, heart rate, mood, and appetite.

Hysterectomy: The surgical removal of the uterus. In some cases, the ovaries are removed as well.

Insomnia: Disturbances in a person's sleep pattern, such as not being able to fall asleep or waking after only a few hours and being unable to fall asleep again.

Menopause: The time when a woman hasn't menstruated for 12 months.

Metabolism: The chemical processes in the body that convert food into usable energy.

Nootropic: A substance that stimulates and supports brain function.

Oophorectomy: The surgical removal of the ovaries.

Osteopenia: The loss of bone density that tends to occur in people older than 50. Although the bones are less dense, the condition hasn't progressed to osteoporosis.

Osteoporosis: A treatable disease characterized by low bone mineral density, low bone strength, and low bone mass, with an increased risk of bone fractures.

Perimenopause: The time when the ovaries gradually stop thWe production of hormones.

Premenstrual syndrome (PMS): Various symptoms that some women experience before their period starts each month. The symptoms include irritability, bloating, and breast tenderness.

Progesterone: A female hormone whose primary role is enabling pregnancy.

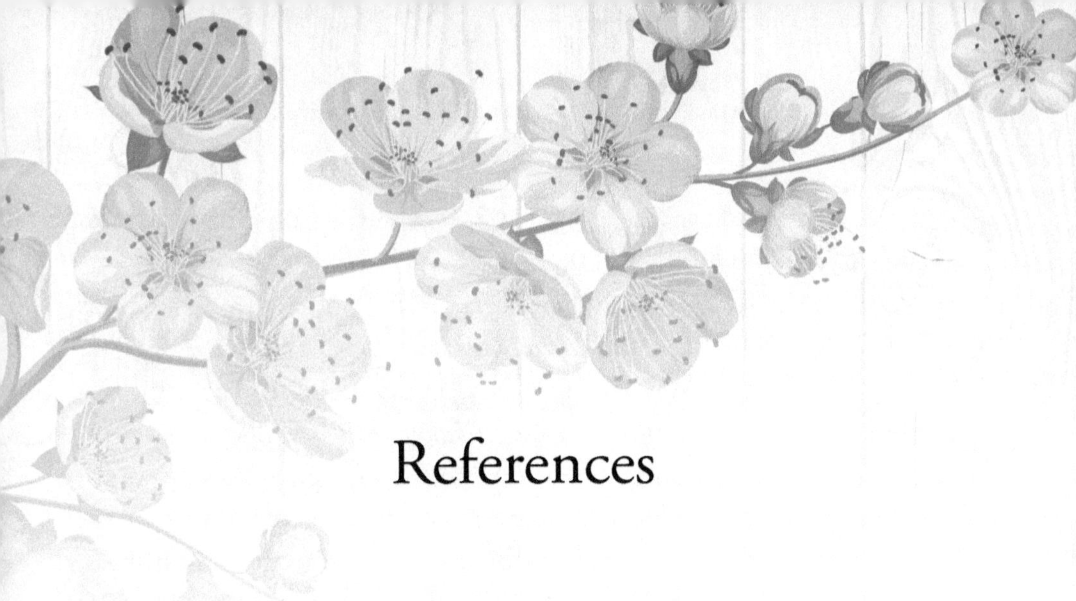

References

Alexander, H. (2021, March 24). *8 foods that impact stress.* MD Anderson Cancer Center, University of Texas. https://www.mdanderson.org/cancerwise/8-foods-that-impact-stress.h00-159459267.html

Allo Health. (2023, August 31). *Ginseng: A natural way to improve memory.* https://www.allohealth.care/healthfeed/medicine/ginseng-for-memory

Alloy. (2023, May 11). *What women need to know about the link between collagen and estrogen.* https://www.myalloy.com/blog/what-women-need-to-know-about-the-link-between-collagen-and-estrogen

Asp, K. (2023, January 26). *Natural ways to cope with hot flashes and night sweats.* Everyday Health. https://www.everydayhealth.com/menopause/natural-ways-manage-menopause-hot-flashes-night-sweats/

Bacopa—uses, side effects, and more. (n.d.). WebMD. https://www.webmd.com/vitamins/ai/ingredientmono-761/bacopa

Bailey, T. G., Cable, N. T., Aziz, N., Dobson, R., Sprung, V. S., Low, D. A., & Jones, H. (2016). Exercise training reduces the frequency of menopausal hot flushes by improving thermoregulatory

control. *Menopause, 23*(7), 708–718. https://doi.org/10.1097/
GME.0000000000000625

Baker, F. C., Siboza, F., & Fuller, A. (2020). Temperature regulation
in women: Effects of the menstrual cycle. *Temperature, 7*(3),
1–37. https://doi.org/10.1080/23328940.2020.1735927

Banbury, T. (n.d.). *Basil essential oil: For memory and concentration.* Mecklenburg Extension Master Gardener Volunteers of
Mecklenberg County. https://www.mastergardenersmecklen-
burg.org/basil-essential-oil-for-memory--concentration.html

Barraclough, A. (2023, October 10). *How gut health can support symptoms
of the menopause.* Women's Health. https://www.womenshealth-
mag.com/uk/food/a45481427/menopause-and-gut-health/

Barazzoni, R., Gortan Cappellari, G., Ragni, M., & Nisoli, E. (2018).
Insulin resistance in obesity: An overview of fundamental alterations. *Eating and Weight Disorders – Studies on Anorexia,
Bulimia and Obesity, 23*(2), 149–157. https://doi.org/10.1007/
s40519-018-0481-6=

Ditzlmüller, L. (2023, May 16). *Lust instead of frustration: Simple exercises and tips to increase libido.* L'officiel. https://www.lofficieli-
biza.com/soul-spirituality/pleasure-instead-of-frustration-sim-
ple-exercises-and-tips-to-increase-libido

18 sneaky names for sugar. (n.d.). Progressive Health. https://www.pro-
gressivehealth.com/sneaky-names-for-sugar.htm

11 supplements for menopause. (n.d.). WebMD. https://www.webmd.
com/menopause/ss/slideshow-menopause

Epel, E. S., McEwen, B., Seeman, T., Matthews, K., Castellazzo,
G., Brownell, K. D., Bell, J., & Ickovics, J. R. (2000).
Stress and body shape: Stress-induced cortisol secre-
tion Is consistently greater among women with central
fat. *Psychosomatic Medicine, 62*(5), 623–632. https://doi.
org/10.1097/00006842-200009000-00005

Eure, M. A. (2023, October 24). *How your sex life changes*

after 60. Verywell Health. https://www.verywellhealth.com/sex-after-sixty-2966815

5 points in CBT to improve a couple's sex life. (203, October 9). Onebright. https://onebright.com/advice-hub/news/5-points-in-cbt-to-improve-a-couples-sex-life/

Fletcher, J. (202, October 4). *How to use 4-7-8 breathig* for anxity. Medical News Today. https://www.medicalnewstoday.com/articles/324417

Fletcher, J. (2022, March 28). *Ginger:* Uses, benefits, and nutrition. Medical News Today. https://www.medicalnewstoday.com/articles/265990

Ford, H. C. (2023, July 12). *Sex after 60? You need to know about STD prevention.* Healthy Balance, UVA Health. https://blog.uva-health.com/2023/07/12/sex-after-60-prevent-std-tips

Frey, M. (2021, October 11). T *he health benefits ofbasil.* Verywell Fit. https://www.verywellfit.com/basil-nutrition-facts-calories-carbs-and-health-benefits-4178775

Frey, M. (2022a, March 28). *Your complete guide to weight loss pills and supplements.* Verywell Fit. https://www.verywellfit.com/supplements-and-diet-pills-to-lose-weight-3495602

Frey, M. (2022b, October 24). *The health benefits of rosemary.* Verywell Fit. https://www.verywellfit.com/rosemary-health-benefits-4587436

Garma, J. (2022, February 28). *Will your belly fat cause cancer?* GarmaOnHealth. https://garmaonhealth.com/belly-fat-can-cause-cancer/

Ghoshal, M. (2022, February 2). *Treatments for menopause symptoms: Prescription, Natural Remedies, and More.* Healthline. https://www.healthline.com/health/menopause/treatments

Gingrasso, A. (2022, April 1). *Good bacteria for your gut.* Mayo Clinic Health System. https://www.

mayoclinichealthsystem.org/hometown-health/ speaking-of-health/good-bacteria-for-your-gut

Goldstein, J. M. (2021, November 3). *Menopause and memory: Know the facts*. Harvard Health Publishing. https://www.health.harvard.edu/blog/ menopause-and-memory-know-the-facts-202111032630

Golen, T. G., & Ricciotti, H. (2021, July 1). *Does exercise really boost energy levels?* Harvard Health Publishing. https://www.health.harvard.edu/exercise-and-fitness/ does-exercise-really-boost-energy-levels

Gordon, J. L., & Girdler, S. S. (2014). Hormone replacement therapy in the treatment of perimenopausal depression. *Current Psychiatry Reports*, *16*(12), 517. https://doi.org/10.1007/ s11920-014-0517-1

Gotter, A. (2023, April 25). *What you should know about chemical peels*. Healthline. https://www.healthline.com/health/chemical-peels

Graedon, J. (2017, November 5). *Licorice to lower libido is risky*. The People's Pharmacy. https://www.peoplespharmacy.com/ articles/licorice-to-lower-libido-is-risky

Grant, P. (2010). Spearmint herbal tea has significant anti-androgen effects in polycystic ovarian syndrome. A randomized controlled trial. *Phytotherapy Research*, *24*(2), 186–188. https:// doi.org/10.1002/ptr.2900

Griffin, R. M. (n.d.). *Which type of estrogen hormone therapy is right for you?* WebMD. https://www.webmd.com/menopause/ which-type-of-estrogen-hormone-therapy-is-right-for-you

Ha, M.-S., Kim, J.-H., Kim, Y.-S., & Kim, D.-Y. (2018). Effects of aquarobic exercise and burdock intake on serum blood lipids and vascular elasticity in Korean elderly women. *Experimental Gerontology*, *101*, 63–68. https://doi.org/10.1016/j. exger.2017.11.005

References

Horny goat weed. (n.d.). MedlinePlus. https://medlineplus.gov/druginfo/natural/699.html

Horny goat weed – uses, side effects, and more. (n.d.). WebMD. https://www.webmd.com/vitamins/ai/ingredientmono-699/horny-goat-weed

The importance of Kegel exercises for menopausal women. (2019, September 7). Pericoach. https://www.pericoach.com/2016/11/08/importance-kegel-exercises-menopausal-women/

Krans, B. (2018, June 15). *Dermabrasion.* Healthline. https://www.healthline.com/health/dermabrasion

Kubala, J. (2023, March 8). *What is collagen, and what is it good for?* Healthline. https://www.healthline.com/nutrition/collagen

Lang, A. (2023, August 7). *10 natural ways to balance your hormones.* Healthline. https://www.healthline.com/nutrition/balance-hormones

Mayo Clinic. (2021a, September 17). *Vaginal atrophy: Diagnosis and treatment.* https://www.mayoclinic.org/diseases-conditions/vaginal-atrophy/diagnosis-treatment/drc-20352294

Mayo Clinic. (2021b, September 17). *Vaginal atrophy: Symptoms and causes.* https://www.mayoclinic.org/diseases-conditions/vaginal-atrophy/symptoms-causes/syc-20352288

Mayo Clinic. (2022, October 11). *Mindfulness exercises.* https://www.mayoclinic.org/healthy-lifestyle/consumer-health/in-depth/mindfulness-exercises/art-20046356

Mayo Clinic. (2023a, April 6). *Sleep apnea.* https://www.mayoclinic.org/diseases-conditions/sleep-apnea/symptoms-causes/syc-20377631

Summer, J., & Cotliar, D. (2023, October 25). *Can binaural beats help you fall asleep?* Sleep Foundation. https://www.sleepfoundation.org/noise-and-sleep/binaural-beats

Petre, A. (2023a, February 1). *7 aphrodisiac foods that boost your*

libido. Healthline. https://www.healthline.com/nutrition/
aphrodisiac-foods

Petre, A. (2023b, July 25). *Are goitrogens in foods harmful?* Healthline.
https://www.healthline.com/nutrition/goitrogens-in-foods

Trend Health. (2020, November 12). *5 major hair stimulators for hair growth.* https://www.trendhealth.
org/5-major-hair-stimulators-for-hair-growth/

Uebel-von Sandersleben, H., Rothenberger, A., Albrecht, B.,
Rothenberger, L. G., Klement, S., & Bock, N. (2014). Ginkgo
biloba Extract EGb 761® in children with ADHD. *Zeitschrift
Für Kinder- Und Jugendpsychiatrie Und Psychotherapie, 42*(5),
337–347. https://doi.org/10.1024/1422-4917/a000309

Van De Walle, G. (2021, May 18). Healthline. https://www.healthline.
com/nutrition/weight-loss-stages *The different stages of losing
weight: Fat loss vs. weight loss.*

Van De Walle, G., & Lamoreux, K. (2023, March 31). *7 science-backed
health benefits of* Rhodiola rosea. Healthline. https://www.
healthline.com/nutrition/rhodiola-rosea

Wattanathorn, J., Mator, L., Muchimapura, S., Tongun, T., Pasuriwong,
O., Piyawatkul, N., Yimtae, K., Sripanidkulchai, B., &
Singkhoraard, J. (2008). Positive modulation of cognition and
mood in the healthy elderly volunteer following the administration of *Centella asiatica. Journal of Ethnopharmacology,
116*(2), 325–332. https://doi.org/10.1016/j.jep.2007.11.038

WebMD. *The emotional roller coaster of menopause.* (2022,
October 6). https://www.webmd.com/menopause/
emotional-roller-coaster

Weight gain: Symptoms, causes, and when to see your doctor. (n.d.). 1MD
Nutrition. https://1md.org/health-guide/heart/symptoms/
weight-gain

Weiss, S. I. (2018, August 27). *5 easy tantra techniques for a serious sexual energy boost*. Well+Good. https://www.wellandgood. com/5-easy-tantra-techniques-for-better-sex/

What are pelvic floor exercises? (2023, November 23). National Health Service. https://www.nhs.uk/common-health-questions/ lifestyle/what-are-pelvic-floor-exercises/

What is a one stitch facelift and how does it work? (2023, April 14). Nourish Your Glow. https://www.nourishyourglow.com/04/ what-is-a-one-stitch-facelift-and-how-does-it-work/

Whelan, C. (2019, August 29). *Skin elasticity: 13 ways to improve it*. Healthline. https://www.healthline.com/health/ beauty-skin-care/skin-elasticity

Wild yam. (n.d.). MedicineNet. https://www.medicinenet.com/wild_ yam/article.htm

Wszelaki, M. (2019, February 6). *How to reduce inflammation fast (and help your hormones, too)*. Hormones & Balance. https://hormonesbalance.com/articles/how-to-reduce-inflammation-fast/

Yadav, U. C. S., & Baquer, N. Z. (2013). Pharmacological effects of *Trigonella foenum-graecum* L. in health and disease. *Pharmaceutical Biology*, *52*(2), 243–254. https://doi.org/10.3 109/13880209.2013.826247

Zelman, K. M. (2008, February 3). *Chocolate's dark secret*. WebMD. https://www.webmd.com/sex-relationships/features/ chocolate-answers

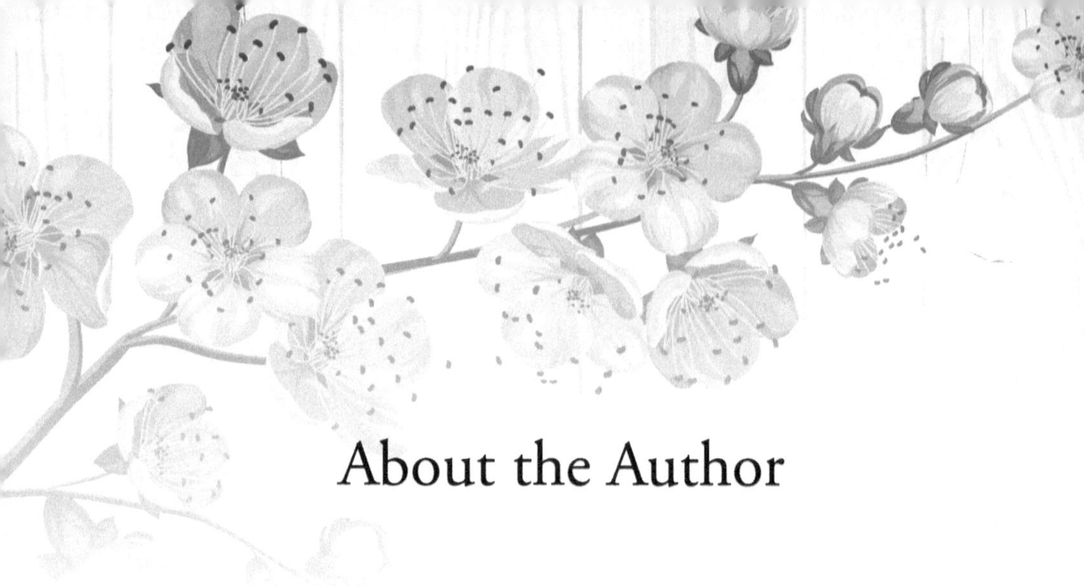

About the Author

Cecilia Baumann is an author with a love for all things spiritual. Cecilia is a proud pet parent to a black and white dog and two mischievous cats who keep her on her toes. Cecilia enjoys exploring the world of tarot, candles, and crystals when she's not tending to her furry friends.

Cecilia is also an avid traveler with a long list of destinations she would love to visit. Whether hiking through the mountains or camping in the great outdoors, Cecilia is always up for an adventure. These days, she prefers RV glamping to tent camping, but she still loves the thrill of sleeping under the stars.

And as you have probably guessed, she is also traveling this menopausal journey, looking for natural solutions to this natural problem and learning along the way.

To find out more about the author, you can go to her website
https://jdsherwood.com

Or the publisher's website
https://sherwoodpublications.com